The Light Inside The Shadow
An Anthology of Works by BlueBoard Members

The Light Inside The Shadow
An Anthology of Works by BlueBoard Members

Members of the BlueBoard Online Mental Health Forum
Edited by Julia Reynolds, Joanne Allen and Michelle Anderson

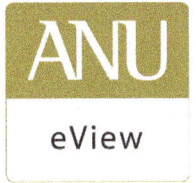

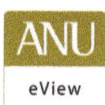

Published by ANU eView
The Australian National University
Canberra ACT 0200, Australia
Email: enquiries.eview@anu.edu.au
This title is also available online at http://eview.anu.edu.au

---

National Library of Australia Cataloguing-in-Publication entry

Title: The light inside the shadow : an anthology of works by BlueBoard members / edited by Julia Reynolds, Joanne Allen and Michelle Anderson.

ISBN: 9781921934155 (paperback) 9781921934162 (ebook)

Subjects: Australian poetry--21st century--Collections.

Other Authors/Contributors:
           Reynolds, Julia, editor.
           Allen, Joanne, editor.
           Anderson, Michelle, editor.

Dewey Number: A821.4

All rights reserved. No part of this publication may be reproduced, stored in a retrieval system or transmitted in any form or by any means, electronic, mechanical, photocopying or otherwise, without the prior permission of the publisher.

All images courtesy of individual contributors

Cover image: Flowers of the Future (creative)

This edition © 2013 ANU eView

Contents

Foreword (Kathleen Griffiths) xi
Preface (Silenus) xiii
Author Statements xv
Editors' Notes xvii

INSIDE THE SHADOW

Darkness

Tears (snowy) 3
No Light Without Darkness (4rensicDJ) 4
Deepression (Silenus) 5
Sinking (MissingLink) 6
Sinking Deeper (GonePirate) 7
We see it shades of red and rust (unlucky?) 8
Inside Depression (creative) 9
darkness reigns (Miseries company) 10
stuck in depression (stressbunny) 11
Ward 4.2 (MissingLink) 13
Not today (squarepeg) 14
Waters (GonePirate) 15
what happens when we are forsaken (Miseries company) 16
Pieces of Mind (GonePirate) 17
what is day (Miseries company) 18
why oh why (Miseries company) 18
The depressed human condition (4rensicDJ) 19
Broken (GonePirate) 20
anger horror pain (Miseries company) 21

The Icarus Flight

Hypo Mania (snowy) 23
If mania is red (Fighter4ever) 24
the ride of my life (GonePirate) 25
The only colour left is blue... (Try2Fly) 26
Fly (GonePirate) 27
Eternal struggle (GonePirate) 29

THE JOURNEY

Me, Myself

Mind Apart (snowy)..33
A life sentence (MissUpNDown) 34
racing, pacing (squarepeg) 35
Wish I'd Never Loved You...... (BipolarBear) 36
I never wanted these problems (GonePirate) 38
I AM (Overtheedge)..40
Ventriloquist Poetry (MissingLink) 41
My Teenage Torture (4rensicDJ) 42
Removing the Mask (GonePIrate).....................................44
rejection (GonePirate) 45
Dah Deh (MissingLink)..46
a guide in the night (GonePirate) 47
If someone would care to walk through the door (Miseries company).....49
Method to my madness (GonePirate) 50
I hurt so bad (Miseries company) 51
Beautiful Dreamer (creative) 52
Recrimination (MissingLink) 53
Letter to myself (creative) 54
Letter to Myself (4rensicDJ) 55
Letter to my 16-year-old self (4rensicDJ) 56

Companions

The Eyes (snowy)..59
He feels them again (unlucky?) 60
You got me (spinningtop17) 61
My Parasitic Twin (MissingLink) 62
Hydra: A Poem for People With Voices in their Heads (4rensicDJ).......64
Visiting Hour (MissingLink)...65
Trapped—A Story about Mental Illness (4rensicDJ) 66
My Curse (Gone Pirate) 70
Rats (MissingLink) 71
The Dog (4rensicDJ) 72
What This Does (4rensicDJ)..73

Living in the World

Mind Trap (snowy) 77
Without Hesitation (creative) 78
My whole philosophy in life is this (GonePirate). 79
the wanderer (GonePirate) 80
we fade from vision (Miseries Company) 81
why is it we can never just be (GonePirate) 83
Another Time and Space (creative) 86
Paddling Back (MissingLink) 87
When I was a child (stressbunny) 88
Absent Father (MissingLink) 89
I miss you (GonePirate) 90

THE LIGHT INSIDE

Brain in a Box (snowy) 93
Baby Squeigh (Squeigh) 94
I am the victim (Newleaf) 95
Failure (TheBeautifulBlueButterfly) 96
The Taste Of Life (Silenus) 97
Middle Age (MissingLink) 98
Moonbathers (creative) 99
Nowhere to hide (creative) 100
You Were There – My Story (Overtheedge) 101
A true story (creative) 103
The Beautiful Blue Butterfly (TheBeautifulBlueButterfly) 104
Joy Ride (4rensicDJ) 105
Notice me? (squarepeg) 106
To those who watch on (stressbunny) 107
To You Who Has Never Known Depression, This Is My Gift (Silenus) 108
Mental Illness: The Butterfly's Thoughts (TheBeautifulBlueButterfly) 113
Stigma (creative) 114
yesterday, today, tomorrow (creative) 115
Eight Legs, Silk, Water and Light (Silenus) 116
A Poem (creative) 117
Reincarnated (GonePirate) 118
Jack was a homeless man (creative) 120

Like strands of wool on a crocheted quilt we provide a net for each other from the abyss of unacknowledgement. We do this with our shared understanding and life experience.

(Chalice)

Foreword

When I first decided to establish BlueBoard I imagined a safe, supportive caring online space where consumers and carers with lived experience of depression could create a community to share their experiences and expertise, understand that they were not alone, and seek help and provide it to others. This would be a place which transcended geographical boundaries and where members could share both the individuality and the universality of their experiences.

In this anthology of creative works, BlueBoard members impart these experiences in a form which is accessible to a wider audience. Consistent with its original aims, BlueBoard members have created a culture of empowerment on the Board and out of that empowerment has emerged a work that will resonate with fellow consumers.

For those who are not consumers but who are brave enough to engage with the work with their eyes open, the anthology will provide a glimpse of a world inhabited by the strongest of unsung warriors who fight an insidious foe with courage and tenacity while engaging with the enemy with the very part of their body which is wounded. By not closing your eyes, you lighten the warrior's load. It is as simple – and as difficult – as that.

I congratulate Silenus for proposing this project, the editors for their work in assembling the anthology, and the authors and artists on their paintings, poems and writings and for their willingness to share their experiences with others. I wish the authors and their fellow BlueBoard members all the light that they can find. I thank the BlueBoard management and moderators for their tireless and dedicated work over many years in maintaining the safe and supportive community that is BlueBoard. Last but not least, I thank you the reader who by keeping your eyes and heart open can ease the load of the BlueBoard warriors and their fellow consumers who seek the light inside the shadow.

Kathleen Griffiths
BlueBoard Director
December, 2013.

Preface

Silenus

This book, an anthology of creative works by members of BlueBoard, is both a sombre lamentation and a joyous celebration of the various conditions that society calls "mental illness" but which we call normal life. Through the medium of creative expression, the contributors to this book have communicated in their own unique and wonderful ways what it is like to live with and experience such conditions as bipolar, depression, anxiety, eating disorders and the like.

Perhaps more than anything, though, these creative works are stuttering steps along our own paths toward a greater understanding of that which we live and breathe every single day. By expressing what our heads and our hearts experience, we do ourselves a great service, expanding our self-knowledge and sharing it with others. It is one of my greatest wishes that, like me, you – the reader of this book – are touched and engaged by our stories.

To my mind, the "disability" that we suffer from as mental health consumers stems not just from the occasional or permanent limitation of our faculties, but from the disconnect between us and society. Society is a human construct, a one size fits all organisation of its many members. It does a fantastic job of dealing with the near-infinite diversity of human beings and the human condition, but when faced with people who suffer from an illness that cannot easily be seen, society is sometimes found wanting. It is alas still in need of developing a greater understanding and de-stigmatisation of those of us who fit outside the definition of good mental health.

I am very grateful that society supports us where our disabilities affect our capacity to support ourselves, but imagine how much better our state of mind and our feelings of self worth would be if society could find a way to utilise our strengths and foster understanding between us all. Much of the stress, pressure, anxiety and trauma associated with having mental health issues could then be transformed to understanding, support, love and hope – in fact all of the wonderful positive qualities that I have found on the BlueBoard forum. We have much to offer society, given the opportunity to do so.

I would wish for this societal disconnect to be changed, through a continual dialogue between "us" and "them". Through that dialogue, we will over time come to realise that there is no us and them at all, only an inclusive and harmonious whole where we each can benefit from the other. This book, for me, is an attempt to build a bridge of understanding and communication between those who have experienced mental health issues and those who have not. It is also a message of hope and understanding from sufferers to their fellows.

So please, dear reader, join us in a celebration of the diversity of the human condition. There's no telling how far down the rabbit hole it goes…

Author Statements

snowy

I don't have words like the others so I use my pencil. The red ball in these drawings represents my mind/ brain, the waves rushing around it are my moods, the continual cycle that carves and shapes with all the power of the ocean.

Drawing is a way of expressing mood and emotion, especially during the times when even simple conversation is beyond reach.

Silenus

I posted four poems for this book, in an attempt to convey the highs and lows of my life with bipolar. My heartfelt hope for this compilation of creative works is that it reaches out and connects with people from all walks of life.

Life is a journey, irrespective of whether one has mental health issues or not. My journey has taught me that my bipolar is an integral part of me – part gift, part curse. The poems I have written are an attempt to explore and make sense of things inasmuch as that is possible. I hope that they communicate that it is possible to accept mental health issues, learn to live with them, and even learn to thrive with them, by embracing both the crushing negatives and the soaring positives as a disharmonious but glorious part of a greater whole.

Missing Link

I'm hoping this book will give people a deeper understanding of mental health from a creative perspective.

Squeigh

I hope this book gives people strength and hope to get through the tough times, and realise that no matter what you are not alone and together we fight for our freedom.

TheBeautifulBlueButterfly

I have written/posted both these poems in the hope of creating awareness of the day to day struggle and experience that bipolar and other mental health sufferers go through. I would also like to point out that I have tried hard to put a positive spin on my poetry to provide hope, while at the same time shining light on the reality of mental illness.

My aim is to make this roller coaster ride as easy as possible.

Editors' Notes

BlueBoard members create a very special space. It is constantly changing and being reinvented, but the space has a solid centre – the respectful sharing of lived experience by its anonymous members.

Sharing on BlueBoard takes many forms. Members can witness the experience of others by viewing the images and text that they have posted. Members may also share their own experiences through writing posts to other members and contributing poetry, short stories, essays and visual images.

During a particularly creative period on BlueBoard, Silenus suggested that these creative works could be published as a book. The idea blossomed and BlueBoard members anonymously contributed the works and the title for this book.

In order to protect privacy, BlueBoard members do not use real names and in this book, authors and artists are referred to by their BlueBoard usernames. These usernames are given in brackets after the title of each work.

As editors, we intervened as little as possible with the material. Our main task was to structure the work using themes that emerged from our reading of the material. We also provided proof-reading and liaised with the publisher.

It has been a great privilege to work on this book. We hope that you will be inspired, deeply moved and enriched by these works.

Inside the Shadow

Darkness

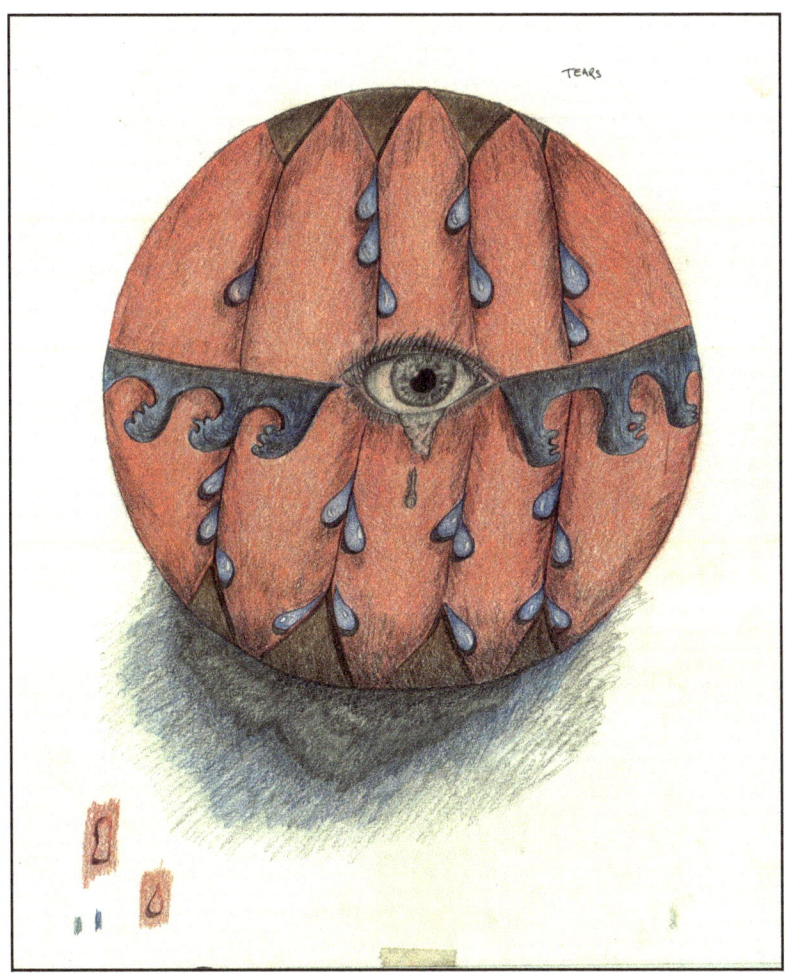

Tears (snowy)

My mind can weep for days, weeks, months. Crying for lost dreams, damage done, to say goodbye, the list goes on. Those tears rarely come out of my eyes any more.

The Light Inside the Shadow

No Light Without Darkness (4rensicDJ)

The darkness seeps in,
Engulfing my body in shadow.
Its tendrils wrap themselves around
and grasp onto my happiness.
The darkness pulls back forcefully,
Taking with it,
Hope and light; humanity,
All that is left in me.

It leaves me cold and harsh,
In pain; seeking revenge.
The darkness toys with my thoughts,
Urging me to complete unmentionable things.
My mind resists.
I lift my head,
Stare at the darkness.
I will have my revenge.

Deepression (Silenus)

I lie here now, a useless lump,
Listening to my heart go thump,
My lead blanket holds me trapped,
A premature shroud in which I'm wrapped.
I cannot face the world today,
My inner demons now hold sway,
Rising, an ocean of tears inside,
I am dead to me, my tears uncried.

I know I should escape my room,
My hopes and dreams lie in this tomb,
Unrealised and trapped, just like me,
A mad fool who longs to be free.
But "should" is just another word,
I berate myself for being absurd,
I bang my head with my fist,
No pleasure for this masochist.

I made it to the front door today,
Believing I would be okay,
I reach a hand out for the knob,
I must get out and do my job.
But like so many times before,
I cannot open that front door,
Instead I turn and get undressed,
Fall into bed, a man depressed.

I look in the mirror from time to time,
Practice fake smiles, a happiness mime,
But I never look myself in the eye,
If I see the emptiness I know I'll die.
And who would I smile at anyway?
I'm lone and alone, (and prefer it that way?)
I hate myself for being so weak,
For being this stupid emotionless freak.

I know that this depression will pass,
And I'll be able to get off my ass,
But tell that to my leaden limbs,
To my precious inner light that dims.
This weight for me is an eternity,
I feel condemned to taciturnity,
I am now at my lowest point,
My failures continue to disappoint.

Sinking (MissingLink)

Somewhere the waves
of dreams break.
That inner child screams
and throws
coloured blocks
through the window
as half rainbows
reach spring's end.

My clarity; lays, flat
in a burning desert
of thoughts,
thirsting for inky droplets
to complete my spectrum of light.

Possibilities slowly cease to be.
I stumble,
lost in a labyrinth
of terra incognita.

Sinking Deeper (GonePirate)

deeper and deeper into the abyss
with my arms shackled I am useless
sinking down to the ocean floor
tied with chains to my own anchor
sinking deeper lungs full of air
release it now I do not dare
fighting is all I know how to do
no I cannot live a life like you
not with enemies haunting my every day
lurking behind every smile in every way
villains that fight to disarm me
step into my shoes and you will see
life isn't easy it's a battle a war
against enemies that are so much more
they pinned me down by my ears to the floor
as they let out the merciless roar
these demons they inhabit human skin
and attack me at my weakest when I cannot win
four days of madness they strike me again
enter four months of sadness I fought in vain
these monsters they trapped me locked me away
kept me their prisoner, it was my price to pay
but as I tried to stand they knocked me back down
they rolled me in chains and they spun me round
tied me to an anchor and cast me to the sea
as I sunk beneath waves my breath held tightly
deeper still without blinking
tied to my anchor I'm slowly sinking

The Light Inside the Shadow

We see it shades of red and rust (unlucky?)

we see it shades of red and rust,
so different from this planet blue from dawn to dusk,
do we travel the darkening skies,
do we dare dream of hope and surprise,
is the dream what keeps us going,
are we truly better off knowing,
it's enticingly easy to lie in the gutter,
to dwell on yourself and no other,
wishing,
wanting,
being,
waiting,
for that familiar cold grasp,
to grip you for the last

Darkness

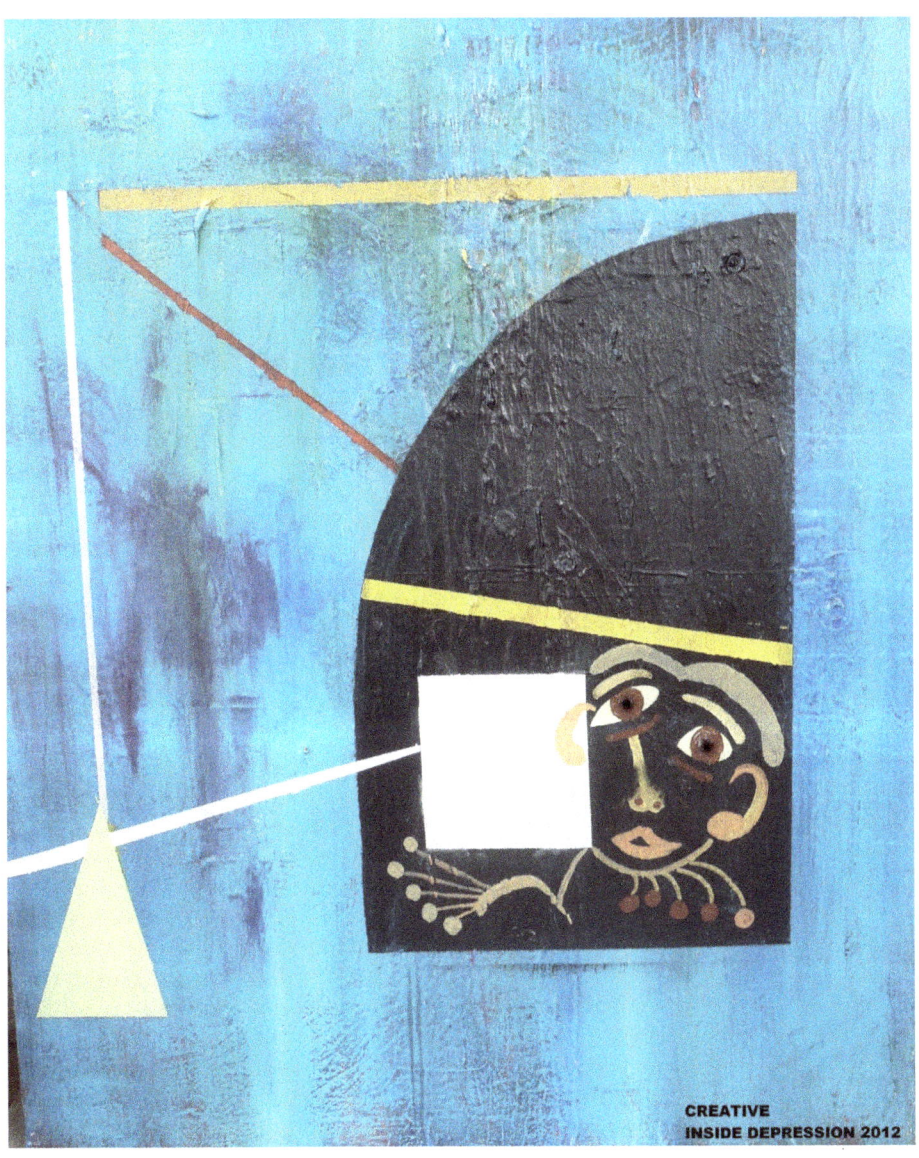

Inside Depression (creative)

The Light Inside the Shadow

darkness reigns (Miseries company)

darkness reigns in the cold bleakness that is my soul, Ragnarok is upon us yet only the mad may see the swarm descending, why must we suffer this travesty this insufferable plague, we do cause we must, we can fight back the storm but can we ever truly see the sun, I look upon the world and weep for what we are and what we shall become, I myself fading, but holding my values and strength high, what my future holds I do not know, will I heal, will I feel, will I be able to trust or care again, will someone breach my pain I know not, but for now I hurt, I hurt for me I hurt for all, I wish everyone happiness, though it is beyond my power to provide such things, we all control our destiny I guess I just tossed mine, maybe it will surface we can only hope to see

stuck in depression (stressbunny)

I'm sitting in soup
it's thick as can be
weighing me down
I am heavy.

I'm stuck in cotton wool
can't breathe at all
wrapped up so tightly
in this cotton wool ball.

I've turned into lead
not impressed might I say
I'd rather be a feather
and see the light of day.

I'm immobilized again
my limbs won't move
so little is done
when I lose my groove.

I'm behind the glass wall
can you see me here?
not getting very far
as I'm in the wrong gear.

I'm heavy as an elephant
not light on my feet
keep going to bed
staying under the sheet.

I'm stuck in depression
can you help me get out
where I'm happy again
with a smile not a pout.
I'm trying to get better
but my life is on hold
I really want a change
but I'm left out in the cold.

The Light Inside the Shadow

I was hoping to be bright
up beat and full of vigor
but I'm dragging the chain
in this mental health rigor.

My psychologist is strange
he seems a little creepy
so I quit at my last appointment
coz I found him way too freaky.

Time is my enemy
sucked me into a vortex
I waste time over-thinking
my poor cerebral cortex!

Out of work and feel a fool
failed again don't you see
I quit my job because I'm sick
It's the pitfalls of anxiety.

Lonely today feeling blue
I'm tired of this game
the test is in staying well
the test is staying sane.

Ward 4.2 (MissingLink)

Twitchy folk, silent folk, babbling folk
shuffle down the corridor
like a chain gang to 'visit' the hospital cafe.
The nurse mouths carefully
Won't that be nice everyone?
Just this morning she said I am listed unsafe
and could not join them yet.
Fuck off then I say and attend a self-esteem group instead.
I action the first step toward it then stop midair
as a lifeless patient is wheeled back to his room
after electro-convulsive therapy.
I ponder how quickly his voluntary signature
translated into a waiver of his rights
I bet he once went for group walks.
Nobody outside has control of the matter
but apparently I am here to regain it.
I nearly lost my tongue but I still have
something to say as I mull over decaf or milo
and pour a safe plastic cup of boiling water.
If I ever see a psychiatrist, I'll be sure to mention it.
Meantime, broken spirited moccasins scuff along a floor
whose history is coated with
bucketfuls of vomit
litres of piss
and the odd dollop of s***e
We all stand around the pool table
watching a game not in play
and try to imagine our local bar.
I take up smoking to pass the eternity of time
absorbing the unkempt garden
wondering how on earth it ever got like this.

The Light Inside the Shadow

Not today (squarepeg)

i cannot think today
not today

i will not feel
not today

i cannot play
not today

i cannot do
not today

i cannot reach out
not today

i cannot reach in
not today

Not today
not today

not today

Waters (GonePirate)

wake me up from my nightmare
wake me up from my sleep
wake me up from this misery
the waters so deep

take away all my innocence
take away all the fire I hold
take away all my willingness
the waters so cold

shine a light in the darkness
shine a light in my cave
shine a light on the shadows
the waters my grave

The Light Inside the Shadow

what happens when we are forsaken (Miseries company)

what happens when we are forsaken, when either by mind or by design we are destined to fall, we put up a strong and valiant fight, but when does it end, does it end, will it end, when do you lay down your sword and let the monsters through, when do you just say you cant fight this war anymore, when do you allow yourself to feel.

when you feel as the mighty titan Atlas, destined to hold the world upon his shoulders for eternity or Prometheus destined to endure his vicious torture everyday forced upon him by the gods, when do you just say the pain is unendurable, when do you just curl up into a ball and just hurt, why must we deal with this pain, maybe it is put on us because we are strong, maybe we just have a glitch in our circuitry, who knows, in the end all make their choices, and in the end we hurt, sometimes there can be seen that light at the end of the tunnel, sometimes just more darkness.

what do I see, well I see no light, just more pain and unending lonesomeness, but I guess that is all my fault, my doing, my torture, so I endure, but will it all crash down, will I crumble under the weight brought to bare upon me, probably, my head hurts all the hurt within attacking full force, all the anger and hate for myself made manifest, tearing, burning, speaking its evil treachery, it is destroying me, can only win so little and lose so much, in the end we do not decide

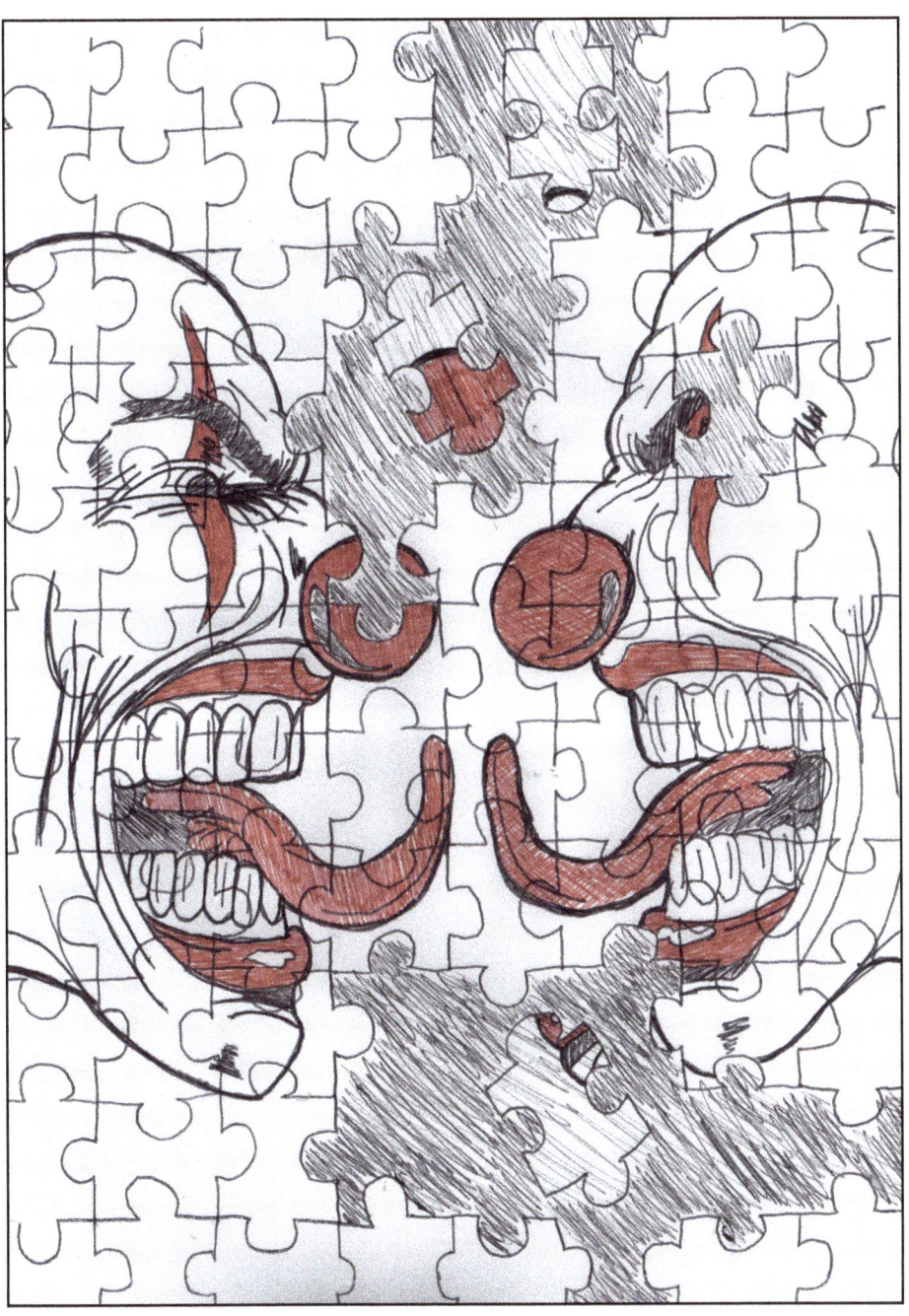

Pieces of Mind (GonePirate)

The Light Inside the Shadow

what is day (Miseries company)

what is day when you live in perpetual night, how can there be light when all you see is darkness, what is laughter when you can barely find a smile, what is joy when you cant enjoy, what are friends when you have only known betrayal, what is love when your heart is broken, what is sadness when you cannot cry, what is pain that is inflicted by mind tearing your body asunder, what is warmth when you live in constant freeze, what is cool when you live in molten rock, why does my skin freeze and my blood boil, why does my heart ache, why does my body weaken, why do I feel, why do I feel like this, why do I care in a one-sided world, why do I see that which burns my eyes, why do I hear that which strains my ears, why do I taste bitter acid, why do I cramp, and why do I sleep and sleep more, it continues no doubt but had to find sense in one so nonsensical

why oh why (Miseries company)

why oh why cant I, why do I hurt, why am I here, why is everything so painful, why do I sit here on the brink of tears but tears do not flow, why is it that I have only ever cried in front of another and very rarely even then, do I seek sympathy, do I seek pity, I think its because I seek comfort, someone to care, someone to tell me this pain is not there, that they will not run, but sadly these are not things that happen not for me, not ever, maybe I do seek those other things I dont know, I just want it all to go away to be clear to see a future of light from this monstrous darkness, this black hole that consumes all, I ride the event horizon of this black hole waiting to be drawn in, wishing it would just go away, wishing there was something of value in me that isnt there, searching my own mental depths for something anything to grab hold of but all thats there is blades and gelatine, I would weep for my loss if I had the heart to, but I dont I just feel like I live in an endless purgatory, walking forever in purgatory along eternity road.

The depressed human condition (4rensicDJ)

The darkness swirls inside,
Desperately trying to find a place to reside.
It plans on sticking around,
And slowly driving me into the ground.
The dog is barking, the cat is scratching,
To my thoughts they are slowly latching,
Onto and I feel weighed down,
I feel as though I'm about to drown.
In a sea of thoughts, horrible things,
And I hate that that's something depression brings.
The world seems to burn,
For more inner peace I yearn,
But there is no light,
I cannot keep up the fight,
I just want to be okay,
And not feel like shit every single day.
I want to be good enough,
Not always having to be tough;
Being strong for myself,
Instead I just sit idly by on the shelf,
Watching other people live their lives,
And this is one of my main deprives.
The feeling of acceptance,
That would make me chase my dog with a vengeance,
The feeling of happiness,
That sometimes just feels so useless.
But I want to be that person,
I have learnt many a lesson.
I don't want more pain,
I want to be sheltered from the rain.
I want the world to make sense,
And finally allow me to survive with no defence.

The Light Inside the Shadow

Broken (GonePirate)

I'm a broken man,
a tortured soul
a shattered mind
trying to be whole

I'm a forgotten plan
the fractured whole
the insane man
out of control

yet I'm the beacon
I'm shining bright
yeah I'm hot and cold
both day and night

I'm the broken soul
the tortured man
the bleeding heart
the bloody hand

I'm the lost wanderer
heading for nowhere
berated by problems
so much it's not fair

broken shattered
****ed in the head
damaged fractured
wishes he was dead

broken beaten
torn apart
lost and defeated
without a heart

anger horror pain (Miseries company)

anger, horror, pain it flows in my veins like rapids pushing my hurting heart, mind and soul beyond breaking point, I have the curse of a strong memory or maybe not memory maybe I just hear, maybe I should wear earmuffs constantly, just so I cant hear, the hearing creates thinking, the thinking creates pain, its not a voluntary action I just take all in even when I do not wish or want to, and the previously mentioned does not help, but I am sure I will hear things such as let it go, get over it, put it aside, but that is not what I do,

I remember all events, I remember every stupid or embarrassing thing I have done while under the influence of drugs or alcohol a big reason to why I do not want anything to do with those poisons anymore, I remember every hurt of any kind that I caused and feel intense guilt for each, I remember every hurt done to me with crystal clarity the ones caused by the person I mentioned previous right at the forefront as there was much, and rather deep wounds,

I remember all and it destroys me, how do you forget, how do you get rid of it, when no-one or nothing has provided happy memories, how do you fight demons that have all the power, how do you fight with no reason no arsenal, yes altering thought patterns may help areas but you can not just forget, you cannot forgive yet accept things that do not work within your values, maybe a little either side is fine but we are talking big time outside my values,

so I see things in black and white, the grey area is limited, and I believe it does not really exist anyway just a question of depth, you are either inside the black or the white just a question of how far, I have wandered into the black zone not as deep as most though, I guess I am deep within the white, alone a lot are on either side of the border probably switching between regularly, but the mid and deep zone of the black area is much more heavily populated, so it is a war I cannot win, I cannot even win a battle, I have strong beliefs I have strong values, but I do not force upon others such things, each person makes their own choice, sadly that leaves me alone, you know what F*** it,

The Icarus Flight

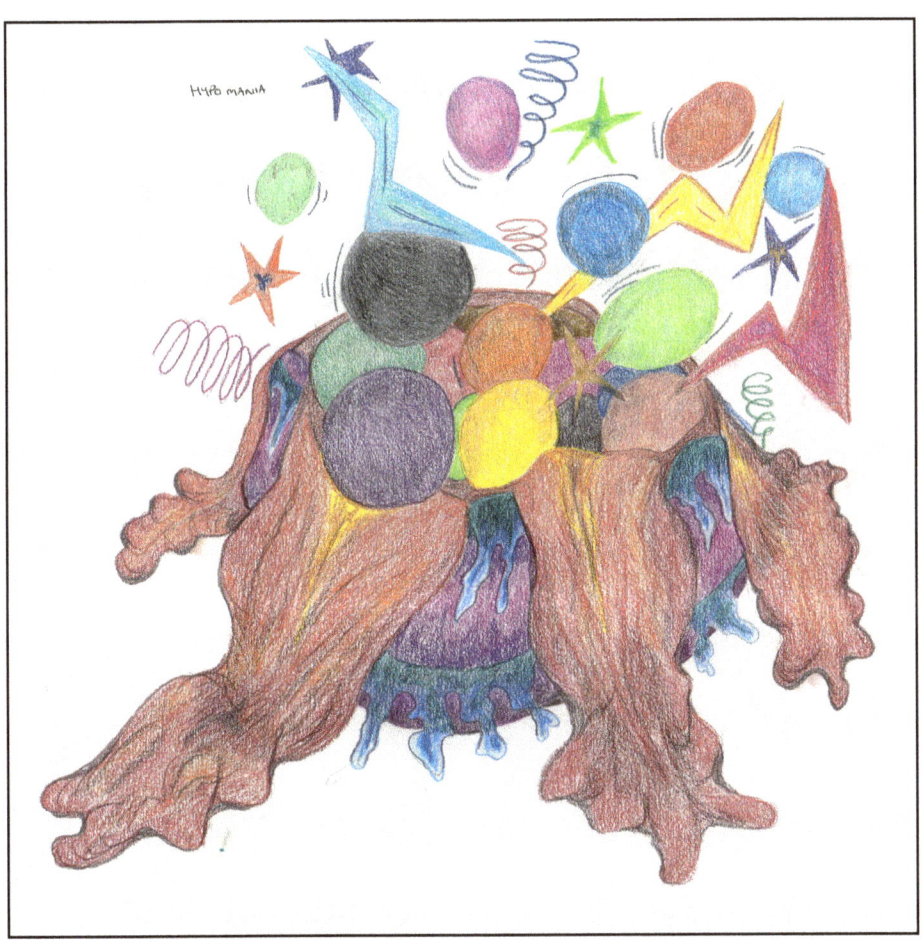

Hypo Mania (snowy)

This is the fun bit of Bipolar – at least for a moment in time. Ideas, energy, plans, just bursting forth, it's like a wonderful party for one, your brain having its own celebration. The world shines, everything looks, feels and sounds better. Then it can change into a paralyzing whirl of ideas, every thought you've ever had. One thought starts before another finishes, a consuming paralyzing hurricane with your mind trapped in the middle.

The Light Inside the Shadow

If mania is red (Fighter4ever)

If mania is red
And depression blue
Then I'm a purple flower
But I'm still of value

the ride of my life (GonePirate)

bipolar as a disease is hard to define
it can attack you both body and mind
so I seek something impossible to find,
Something which is a habit of mine
finding people of a similar mind...

bipolar as a life is hard to define
it's a foe that can attack the mind
and even if you close your eyes
it's something from which you cannot hide
you're just going along for the ride...

The Light Inside the Shadow

The only colour left is blue... (Try2Fly)

Tomorrow wakes but cannot rise
(Lows are dues that pay for highs)
A single tear rolls down each cheek
Trembled lips can hardly speak

Did I just live through a dream
Of rushing thoughts - a gushing stream
Where every rainbow led to gold
All the colours bright and bold

Trusting sunshine follows rain
I slowly push against the pain
Kicking covers from the bed
Fighting demons, wearing lead

One thing that I'm sure is true
The only colour left is blue...

Fly (GonePirate)

I've soared higher than others dare to dream
let out cries louder than others care to scream
I've done all that is expected of me
seen all that there is to see
soared higher than the highest heights
shone brighter than the brighter lights
but burnt out far too quick
and made myself sick, what a prick
I've flown higher than the clouds of the sky
felt so good so free that I could die
and be happy of what I've done
so high I could almost touch the sun
I've done everything I wanted to do
but not what was expected from you
lived by my own terms at my own speed
fuelled by wanting lust and greed
only thinking of what I need
I've flown so high to fall so low
gone so fast to go this slow
crash and burn plummeting
with no last song left to sing
fallen from the sky down to the earth
to crash and sink beneath the surf
drifting deeper underwater still
lost all control and all free will
the murky depths become my home
and twist the beliefs that I have known
alienating me for what I condone
I've sunk deeper into the regret
sinking into the big dark wet
holding tightly to my last breath
patiently waiting for my death
but it never comes no matter how hard I pray
I sink to the ocean floor and deeper in a day
only to find myself on the upwards climb
rock bottom is near impossible to find
ever since that day when I lost my mind
flying so high the depths far beneath me
try as you might you just cannot reach me
never felt so good it was intoxicating

but the depths that haunt me sat in waiting
knowing I cannot fly so high without coming down
my moods fluxuate and change around
I cant explain how feeling so good did so much damage
but if I wasn't flying I couldn't have managed
half of what I've been through in my life
mistakes and trouble chaos and strife
I gave in and took a dive

only dreamers fly into the sky
reaching heights ever so high
even if only to crash and die
never ever to ask why...

Eternal struggle (GonePirate)

I am destined to be alright
but first I must fight
endless through the night
with all of my might
I am destined to fall
to the weight of it all
this endless pain
inside my brain
the eternal struggle
I am destined to fail
weakened and frail
destined to be crushed
if the process is rushed
destined to run
run off into the sun
the eternal struggle
I cannot retort
to this endless thought
that I am not worth the fight
and I won't be alright
not if this can do anything
to attempt to bring
me down to the ground
spin me round and round
till I'm dizzy and dazed
my body unphased
the eternal struggle
but my mind in chains
my body feels the pains
as my mind explains
why suffering runs in my veins
I am destined to die
with this look in my eye
like I meant it all along
dead with a grip on the bong

The Journey

Me, Myself

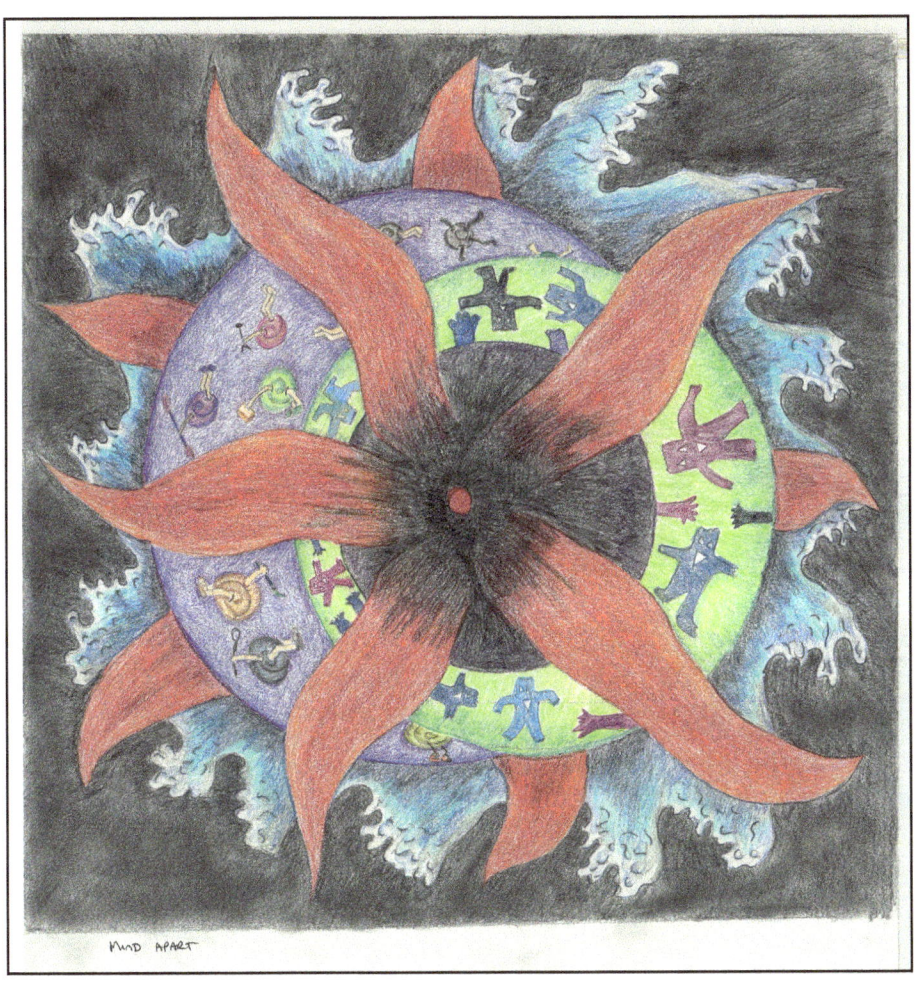

Mind Apart (snowy)

Occasionally, for no obvious reason, my mind just rips apart and all that I am, and all the demons inside me just come spinning, ripping, tearing out of my mind. My mind explodes, I'm lost.

A life sentence (MissUpNDown)

A numbness surrounds her. Her soul feeling flat and lost somewhere deep within. All her emotions laying low, knowing they are there, feeling them itch under the surface, but with no relief.

Her eyes empty as she stares and daydreams of contentment, hoping to one day experience the sense of freedom, freedom from the prison she has created within herself.

Reaching out, cold iron bars stinging her hands, a harsh reminder of the lost identity.

Gripping at the lock, fearing a loss of reality, scared to be discarded from society, with no more than heavy eyes and a damaged heart.

Her soul sees through, but for only a moment, a single tear rolling down her face, her flushed cheek soaking up the little relief, a sign that she is still praying to survive...and to continue to fight.

racing, pacing (squarepeg)

racing, pacing
brewing and stewing
asking, questioning
seeking and searching
thinking, listening
processing and whinging
solution, problems
thoughts and feelings
sensations reeling
way too much thinking
burnout, numbness
screaming and silence
meltdown, shutdown
fractured and splintered
state of mind

The Light Inside the Shadow

Wish I'd Never Loved You...... (BipolarBear)

I guess you'll tell me I already had my chance,
You gave me time,
The choice was mine,
And you'll remind me that you offered me the last dance,
And I refused,
And you turned and left the floor....
Will I be sorry now, forever more?

Up to now I've been looking for a reason,
To make amends,
To try again,
But someone else has taken over in the meantime,
And I've lost the chance,
And I can't believe what a fool I've been....

I waited too long, to tell you how I'm feeling,
I was still getting over the pain of the fall,
Now I've left it too late,
There's no second chances,
And I wish I'd never loved you at all.......

I should've known that you wouldn't wait forever,
You kept calling, I kept stalling,
And she moved in while I was searching for an answer
That I couldn't find,
And you wanted something more,
I'm only sorry now I know the score.

Up to now, I've been searching for a reason,
To make amends,
To try again....
But someone else has taken over in the meantime,
And I've lost the chance,
And I can't believe that I let it go so easy...

I waited too long, to tell you how I'm feeling,
I was still getting over the pain of the fall,
Now I left it too late,
There's no second chances,
And I wish I'd never loved you....

Wish I'd never left you, never lost you, never met you.....
Wish I'd never loved you at all.

Author's note:

I originally penned this piece as a song in my early 20's. At the time it was a lamentation to lost love.... but I've recently seen a deeper meaning in the words that was originally unintended, as I had not been diagnosed with bipolar at the time of writing.

Bipolar has created in me two distinct personalities, the down girl and the up girl, and they don't like each other very much. I now see these two girls battling it out in the song. I hope the meaning translates for others.

The Light Inside the Shadow

I never wanted these problems (GonePirate)

I never wanted these problems,
now I think that I love them,
feel I depend upon them,
as if feeding from them,
but I cannot become them,
so I attempt to stay clear
but it all just reappears in a couple more years
with a few too many beers

With that comes a wave of tears
and overwhelming cheers
a body without thought only instinct steers.
Never wanted to love it,
thought that I was above it.
thoughts about lying dead in a bloodstained coffin.

But I cannot rest,
not with this weight on my chest,
cause when I'm at my best
I must attempt to stress
the importance of being humane

when there ain't nothing left.
And your only choice is to cry out for death.
because I dug too deep in my mother****ing brain.

Left with no more fantasies to entertain,
now I don't feel that sane,
like my life's mundane,
too damn boring and plain,
I'm just circling the drain,
leaves behind a blood stain,
as I split these wigs,
and they paint my kicks
while I light my cigs
and I smoke my twigs,

**** you too cause you ain't that big,
think your so ****ing smart try and solve this shit
bring me back my kid,
get me one more hit,
make me forget this grit
before I throw another fit
and end up lying in a pit
with a hole in my head and a brain full of shit.

Me, Myself

but there ain't no way the world could never take me,
by my own hand maybe
but now never mistake me
I'm not suicidal, I just ****ing hate me
and if I **** this up again I won't hesitate to break me
to ****ing devastate me
snap the **** in half for even thinking he could take me,

but I don't give names
and I don't play games
you ****ing get around like you got no shame
and no I don't blame
no you're not the reason I'm insane
you're just a ****ing name
in the obituaries page
another ****ing lump in a shallow ****ing grave.

and you'll never know when I'm gonna meet ya
but that is when I'll treat ya
to the main ****ing feature,
this is how I will defeat ya,
I'll absorb you and become a brand new creature.

but I'm trying to behave and be a little bit decent,
I haven't hurt a single mother****er as of recent,
and I been seeking psychological treatment.
maybe it's just that I'm in more control than you thinking.
sure I can shift and change in just a blink and,
can lose myself entirely when I start drinking
and I want to bail out because of what I have been thinking
the whole ship is sinking and the world's on the brink man

I just say enough and I throw a little stink and
I pack another cone until its falling out the rim and
I grab the green lighter that I'm holding in my left hand
then choke down my soul through the kink in my s bend.
The world is ****ing poison
and I'm a ****ing dead man.

I AM (Overtheedge)

Am I a person of substance or just a fail,
Am I attractive or just too pale,
Am I intelligent or just deluded,
Am I worthy enough to be included

Am I essential or can just be replaced,
Am I admirable or just a disgrace,
Am I strong or just too broken,
Am I of value or am just a token

Am I funny or just a dummy,
Am I a good parent or a useless mummy,
Am I worthy of love or just indifference,
Am I important or don't mean threepence

Am I wise or just hot air,
Am I compassionate or just don't care,
Am I interesting or just a bore,
Am I warm or really need to thaw

Am I patient or just too short,
Am I virtuous or just don't get caught,
Am I truthful or just live a lie,
Am I truly living or just alive

Am I searching or just cursing,
Am I serious or just rehearsing,
Am I looking or just too blind,
Am I helpful or just unkind

Am I in reality or lost in space,
Am I belonging or just missed the race,
Am I stable or my thoughts just scattered,
Am I worthy or just don't matter

I AM

Ventriloquist Poetry (MissingLink)

The ventriloquism of poetry
has a dizzy, floating effect.

haw haw, guffaw.

Silence mouthpiece while a hand recites
palpable posey.
This automaton pretense
giddies my sense of stability.
Grinning like a stooge's patsy,
I perform only as a sideshow dummy.
So be my backbone and let the sketch continue.
Go on. Applaud, laugh, boo.
My character mumbles balladry
while you puppeteer the next verse with strings.
Alter my rotating habit of circular themes
Up and down
Side to side

(A slapstick pie in the face will fit right here.)
Kasplatch!

Haven't you noticed my lip-synched doggerel
swooning through labyrinths of bone and soft tissue,
pounding your ears each sunrise?
Part of me writes in sleepy fluid-filled loops
but when I'm tipped to one side,
your hand releases its grip and I lose my spine..
At the closing part of the act,
harmony crumples like a heavy curtain
as I tumble to the last line
like some vague, senseless point.

The Light Inside the Shadow

My Teenage Torture (4rensicDJ)

Why do I feel like this?
I feel as if my world is falling apart around me,
Like everyone I love is slowly distancing themselves from me.
I feel as if all I do is give, give, give,
But I never get back,
I live to serve others,
I conform to suit their needs, not my own,
My parents expect me to sit like a good girl,
Never speak,
Never talk back,
Never think for myself.
I rebel more often than not,
Just so somebody knows I exist.
I feel as if my world is falling apart around me,
I have no true friends left,
No one to talk to,
Trust,
Or confide in,
My 'friends' are all chipper, happy, loving,
Making me feel more depressed than usual,
My latest conform is my body,
My body is all I am,
Without it,
I'd be no one.
Sluttiness gets me far,
Gets me noticed,
Gets me loved.
All I wish for is a true friend,
And I will get one,
No matter if I have to kiss, hug, or let my body be...
My body is all I am,
If I was only based on my personality,
I'd be ruined,
Unloved,
More than I am now.
I have been kicked, hit, bitten,
Worse than that,
Called names,
Lied to,
Tricked and betrayed,

Me, Myself

Used.
I feel as if my world is falling apart around me,
I know that I have never been loved,
I know that I never will be,
I think that if I once again conform,
I may eventually fit in
With the people around me,
Finally,
I may be able to be myself,
Let the true me be seen,
However,
I'm scared,
Afraid,
Traumatized.
What if they don't like me?
The real me.
I want to go back to that girl,
The girl before all this,
The girl that stood up for what she believed in,
The girl that didn't care what people thought of her,
The one that wasn't afraid,
Said what she believed,
Was comfortable in her own skin,
And wouldn't take shit from no one.
Why can't I be that girl?
The girl I used to be,
Before the city,
Before the new school,
Before... Before *him*.
I can never be that girl.
The things that have happened recently,
Will haunt me forever,
Never leaving my side,
The big elephant in the room.
Why do I feel like this?
Because I let myself be influenced by others,
Be changed by others,
Be controlled by others.
And that's a fact that will never change,
No matter how hard I try,
It will never change.

The Light Inside the Shadow

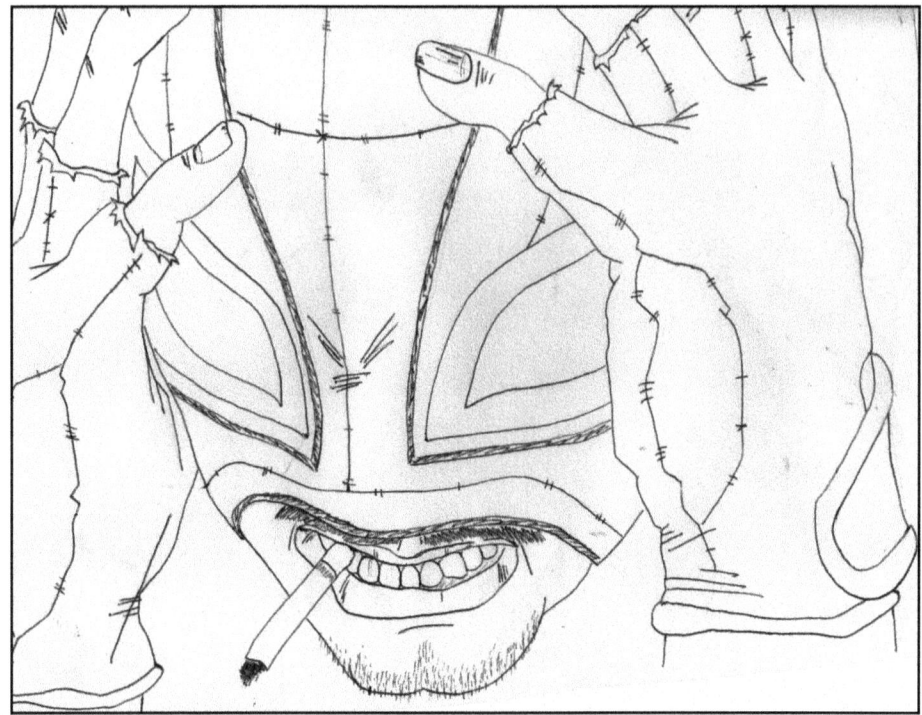

Removing the Mask (GonePirate)

rejection (GonePirate)

every day draws closer to death
I can feel the life running dead
each second draws to my last breath
and I just want to get out of my head
I could pray for days in vain
pray to imaginary friends
if you talk to yourself you're insane
but I feel that just depends
on the perspective with which you stand
staring at my own reflection
slowly extend a hand
then draw it back in with rejection

The Light Inside the Shadow

Dah Deh (MissingLink)

On life support
I'm choking inside of myself
in this world
of silent horror
the tube slipping in
then out
raping my unthought thoughts
my hearing deadened
to the sound
of you being around
blips and bleeps
eternal sleep
wondering how
my next verse
will be fertilized
swimming through wave
after wave of nausea
I drift out with the tide

a guide in the night (GonePirate)

I find myself stuck, I am not moving
as what is real I'm slowly losing
talking speaking found amusing
but incompetent from times abusing
afraid of opening up to be hurt again
afraid to stand out and be my own man
**** my brain it has turned against me
but I feel as if I'm never gonna see
another day or another tomorrow
my own weakness my greatest sorrow
and I know I've said it before
but I'm struggling and something more
I'm drowning trying to catch my breath
as everyday feels closer to death
so I sit alone in a room and doubt
screaming frantically wanting out
drop a beat and I find some peace
draw some dreams until my mind's at ease
but depression creeps on and takes me away
to another place that I cannot say
extend a hand a gesture to follow
take a deep breath through that lump and swallow
follow madness into the mine field
still feeling like I cannot deal
grips like ice this anxious foe
frozen solid my brain runs slow
fly so high just to crash and burn
shoot myself in the foot at every turn
the enemy of my enemy is surely my friend
but my enemy is me so I'm my own end
so I chop up my hopes and mix in my feelings
light up my dreams and I can start dealing
with these issues with overwhelming confidence
something that's missing since I lost my competence
bipolar, depression, anxiety to boot
a mean little bastard in need of a root
with no self esteem and a sad little smile
who just wasted away after a while
once such greatness held up above
so much importance when so much in love

The Light Inside the Shadow

>but everything comes at the direst cost
>what have I become when all love was lost
>mean and twisted despise for them all
>belittling and evil can make you feel small
>but still full of compassion a friend and a dad
>but so far from happiness constantly sad
>seeking upliftment a rise in my mood
>or seeking a lady for something so rude
>anything to take my mind off the fight
>and whatever will guide me off through the night

If someone would care to walk through the door (Miseries company)

if someone would care to walk through the door then it is there but I will not seek that which will just destroy me, and asking that someone would want to walk to let alone through that door is way to much to ask of anyone especially when all they need do is exist and they shall have many falling at their feet, makes me gone, never to ever feel the only thing I have ever desired, so that means my only aspiration is now lost,

so where does that leave me, gone, a wisp of smoke on the air just fading, with but a few words and prose remaining, watching those around pair up and fade away, breaking what little is left of my already straining heart, to lose at love as I have lost at life, we all suffer our pains, my heart once so big and strong, now a fluttery pebble that still feels as deeply, still falls as hard, still wishes as strongly, and is still hit as hard, pierced as deep, hurt as heavily.

and so all that is left for me is to weep for that I have never known, to cry tears of pain that do not matter, to suffer my own torment at failing so completely

in here the poison drips from my lips to the ears of those of heart, outside here I bite my lip, I swallow the poison, for peoples protection, I speak in random niceties, in courtesy, as with my actions, I hold to principles and values that made me the person I was and maybe the person I am, though I may be damaged, fractured as it were I am still the sweet soul, and pure of heart, the mystery, the shadow,

strange that I must be this, a vision an aspiration

Method to my madness (GonePirate)

there's a method to my madness
an eye to the storm
there's a joy within my sadness
wherein I feel the norm
there's a method to my madness
sanity for the insane
there's a goodness to my badness
thought without a brain
there's a method to my madness
a frown within a smile
there's a sorrow to my gladness
which is fatal once in a while
there's a method to my madness
a fire for a light
there's a method to my madness
with no end in sight

I hurt so bad (Miseries company)

I hurt so bad at any given moment, why can it not just leave me be, but I guess if it did then I would be at yet another impasse how to exist, I have no friends, to family I am like a static fixture, to everyone else in the world I am nothing or if I am really lucky an annoyance, why is it so that I must face this insidious bleakness that has no end, I don't know just must deal with it I guess, everyone must face their demons, mine no worse or no stronger than anyone else's, but all I do is look hard seek hard for a reason, some tangible meaning, some reason to keep fighting,

friends I have met here help, but the fantasy can never last and then it is back to being me alone against insurmountable odds, I try, I hold on, I keep searching, but in the end I guess its merely me, just one weak pathetic cowardly loser against something unseen, it is what it is I guess, in the end the only thing I have is me all I have ever had is me, all I will ever have is me, except in a dream world where I can have worth and hope if only for a moment, but the dream world is gone now, no more dreams, no more illusions just pain, hurt, suffering, me alone facing an army descending like a plague of flies.

alone we face the demons, alone we walk upon the scorched earth of war, alone we must fight, no reprieve, no respite, just more battles to face, an endless struggle against our own minds, can we win, unknown

I walk alone within my lifemare for eternity, cause it is all I deserve, because I ask too much, that it was not so, that I could find a reason a means to garner strength, but it is not to be, it is what it is it cannot be helped, sooooooooooooooo cold

The Light Inside the Shadow

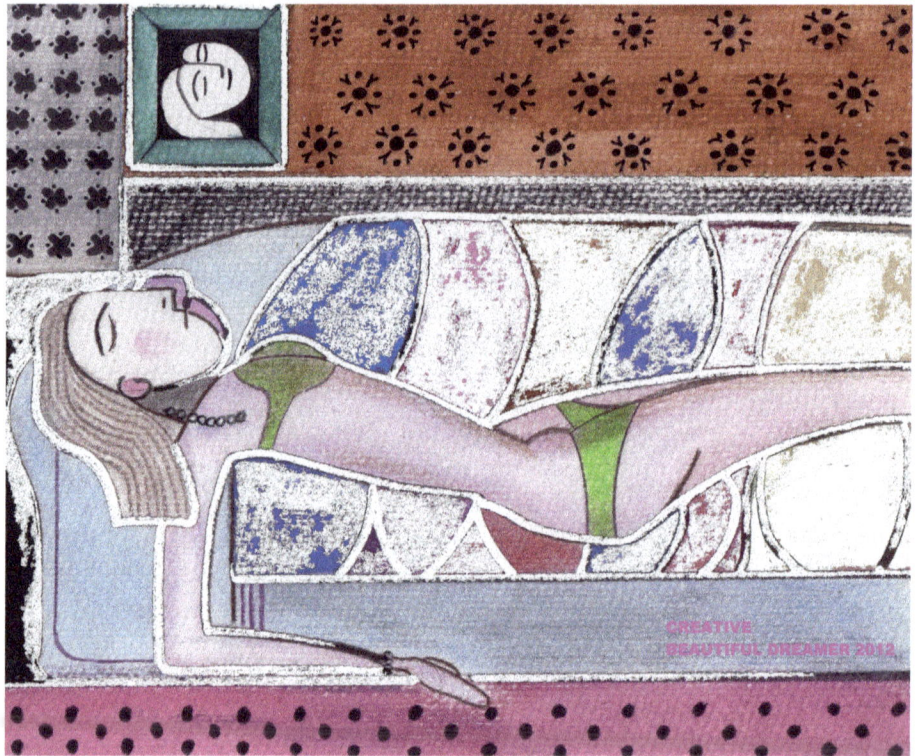

Beautiful Dreamer (creative)

Beautiful dreamer is a watercolour painting inspired by a dream. I have made many versions and variations of this painting the first one was made a few years ago and this is the best version.

Recrimination (MissingLink)

Birds will sing
on the day I deface
gouge
and erase
all memory of this monster,
starting with sinewy arms
snaking round my neck

As I crouch
in the stoning
with my suffering offspring,
at least let me
slice off the heads
of my own toxic hydra

Letter to myself (creative)

What is this thing called mental illness? Do we really have all of the answers? Or are we fumbling in a sea of darkness, where we make up theories and hypotheses as we go? And does this fumbling, that we call knowledge, affect our understanding in our attempt to get closer to the truth?

I suspect that one day, hopefully, we will realize that our idea of a mental illness is highly inadequate. Perhaps then we will see it not as permanent illness but as a temporary disorder. Society will change, stigma will be a thing of the past and we will be able to work on our mental disorder becoming more and more able to cope. This will be possibly because of the social support, now practically non-existent, and because most people will have understood, by necessity, that developing a mental disorder can happen to anyone without discrimination.

We will understand that childhood traumatic experiences make up the great majority of mental disorders, and that trauma is the major cause of mental disorders.

I suspect that as more and more people become sufferers, given that what we call mental illness is increasing, we will have to change our ways.

For now we remain locked in our ignorance and we see some uneven progress. What could speed up the process is knowledge, experience and the development of wisdom. I hope to be able to see this day in my lifetime but I have my doubts.

For now I am part of the currents that bring change and of this I am very proud and this is possible because I have come to understand that the human mind is magical.

Letter to Myself (4rensicDJ)

Dear Deej,

You need to realise your potential. Stop putting yourself down. When others around you tell you something honestly in regards to how wonderful you are, you shut them down and believe they are lying to you. Let them compliment you, let the love they feel for you soak into your veins and never take it for granted as one day, they might not be by your side anymore.

Don't take things personally. If people ignore you or stop being your friend; their problem, not yours. It is not your fault that people don't like you, perhaps it's because you are too good for them, but I know you do not see yourself this way.

If someone messages you and then doesn't reply for an hour; they're probably just busy, so don't take this personally either, although I know your anxiety and lack of self-esteem doesn't help.

You need to realise that you are beautiful and to let people in. People will only try and break your barriers so much, and if you keep turning away, they might turn away themselves and I know you don't want that.

Keep your head up my dear and try to think of things positively. You are actually a much better person than you give yourself credit for, and I cannot wait for the day when you realise that, and when you realise that you are special and you are worth something.

Keep the faith and look to those around you; they are the people that care about you most, so don't push them away, even when times get tough because that is when you'll need them most.

Love, Deej xx

The Light Inside the Shadow

Letter to my 16-year-old self (4rensicDJ)

To my Dear Deej,

I'm writing to you as an 18-year-old version of yourself, so keep in mind that the awesome things I'm about to say are only a couple of years away!

I'll begin with what you think of yourself now.

I know you are struggling with your personal image and trying to pull the girl who you once were back out to show the world... Keep pulling! It pays off! You are struggling with boys like the majority of 16 year old girls do, but don't let this issue worry you...

Yes, you did have a relationship with a d*ck of a guy, but please try and force yourself to remember they aren't all like that, even though I know it's tough to think that sometimes. You've always been closer to guys than girls, and always fitted in with them more, and that keeps going... One of the guys around you will surprise you and confess his love for you, so just be yourself, because that's what he likes. I know it's hard to believe things work out for you in this department, but I'm being honest; and it's fantastic!

You're experimenting with alcohol and rebelling often against your parents... They've always annoyed you with their decisions, but they really were just trying to look out for you... But don't worry, they ease up and you get out of there as soon as year 12 is over...

You are living your dreams, studying the things you wanted at University and you have an awesome guy by your side who accepts you for you and always makes you smile... Cherish him and never let him go.

In regards to your depression; it is still here, but is definitely not as prominent as it is in your mind now. You learn to live and function with it and it becomes bearable. I know that some days you just never want to get out of bed and just give up at school, but persevere; you become stronger because you kept going!

You are one tough cookie and you've been through so much in your short lifetime. There are without a doubt still ups and downs and terrible times when you don't think you can pull your life back from the grips of the dog, but always remember that the people around you love you, and they've stuck with you through everything so far, so they aren't going anywhere!

Just believe in yourself. You choose pretty well, with some exceptions. You're biggest regret will be losing your virginity to that d*ck, but you learn your lessons and wait to see if someone proves they love you first, before you go chasing after pure words...

Good luck my darling, and there is light at the end of your pitch black tunnel.

Love you always,

Your 18 (and legal) old self.

P.S. Just because you are legal now in that regard, doesn't mean you should go throwing yourself around... Wait for that friend that becomes that guy. It will be the best decision you ever made.

Companions

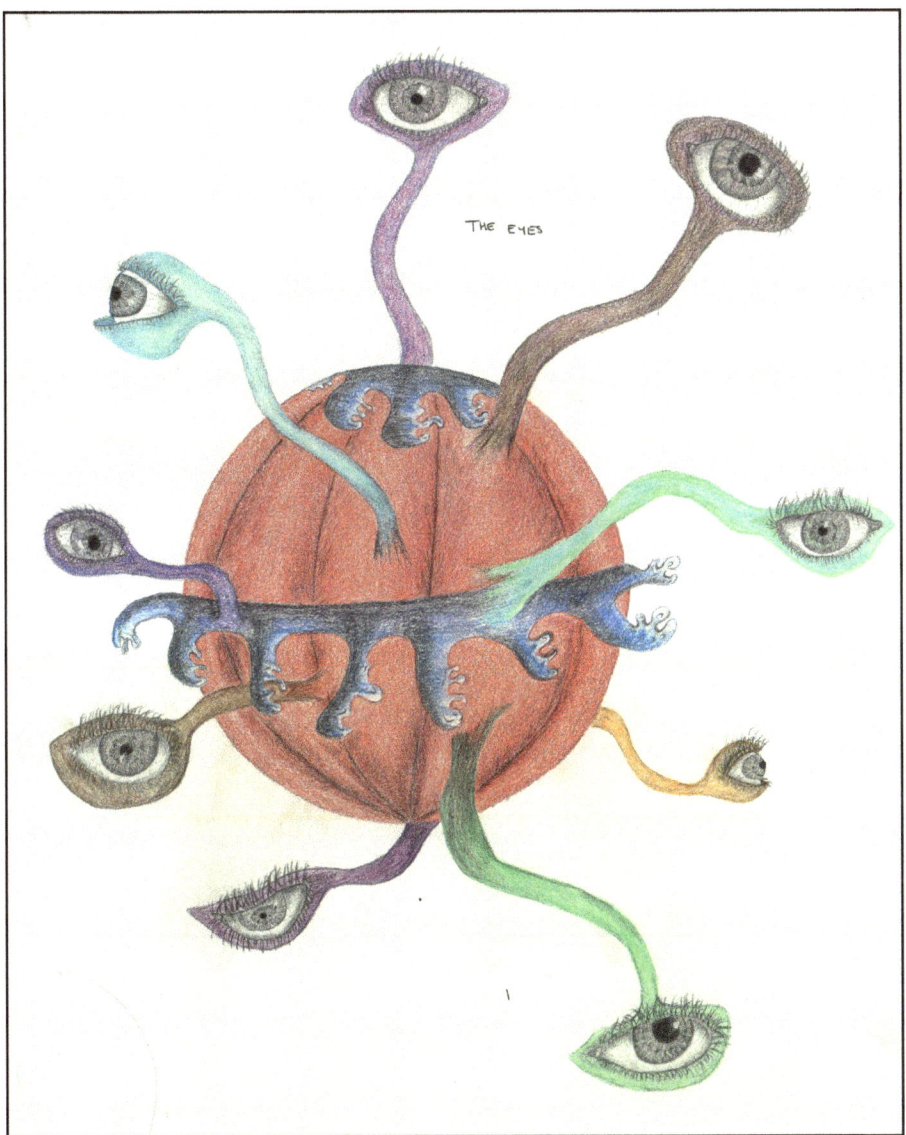

The Eyes (snowy)

Hyper-vigilance is part of bipolar for me, probably the combination of bipolar and trauma working together. I'm aware of all that happens around me, I can't filter out noise and movement. I constantly startle, need to sit with my back to the wall and face the door and so on it goes. It's distressing and limiting. I've worked hard for years to control it but it never really goes away.

The Light Inside the Shadow

He feels them again (unlucky?)

He feels them again, creeping around in his head, the spiders' rough hairy legs scratching, probing, trying to find a hold, their poison dripping into every thought, every feeling, every inch of his being, tainting his very existence.

He tries to scream, tries to let them all know its not him, that he's sorry but he can't, paralyzed and helpless, no one hears.

Alone he sits in his room tears a warm, waxing river coursing down his unshaven face. Alone with the weight of knowing, alone with the fear, alone with those spiders crawling all through his mind, his unwanted companion, his only true friend.

What cruel irony that his torturer must be his final confidant.

You got me (spinningtop17)

Tried so hard to let you go,
To tell myself you're gone,
But you've replaced all that I know,
The person lost, the one I mourn.

I've tried to escape the shackles -
To release your mighty grip,
I struggle and you cackle,
You watch as I fall and slip.

You thief! You took everything that was my own
You have consumed me, yet you want more.
You are here with me, but I still feel so alone,
Feeling so faithless, detached from my core.

You captured my essence in a little black bottle,
You seized my vision, my hearing, and my sanity.
From behind the shadows you revealed a model,
But that girl, she isn't me…

My Parasitic Twin (MissingLink)

I call him Freddy but only to freak villagers out. He doesn't have a name. He just is. When people meet Freddy, their faces contort in morbid horror when they see him protruding awkwardly from my abdomen. His arms and legs wrap round me like a baby monkey. You can run your fingers from his small bottom all the way along the rigid bumps in his spine to the nape of his neck. My Mother believes Freddy's head is my heart and it is only through him that I live. Not the other way round. When I study myself in the mirror, Freddy really does look as if his head has disappeared into my chest. His hands, half holding on are just as easily trying to push his body away so his head will pop out and he'll exclaim, 'Finally!'

The doctor calls me the Autosite, like I'm some mechanic who keeps Freddy the Parasite going. He should be grateful, all things considered. It is my organs that are doing all the work and let's face it; Freddy would not exist without me. I have a hole in my heart due to the extra blood that must pump through his body so he can grow at the same rate as me. I tell Mother this, hoping she will appreciate me more but she won't hear of it and slaps the back of my head instead. 'You dare think you're better than your brother? Who are you to come into this world and put yourself above everyone else? I tell you, your brother says more wise things through his presence than you could ever speak in a lifetime!' She makes me cart an extra basket up the mountain for being so proud and haughty. Freddy's clinging shape wobbles lifelessly as he holds on. 'I'm saying nothing,' is his internal reply as he lets me struggle under the full weight of his body. My mind is flooded with notions of 'but it isn't my fault, it's his!' unsure which of us is doing the thinking.

At home Mother prepares dinner over hot coals. My Father descends from the mountain and kisses us wearily. He is a quiet man. He strokes me after dinner as if I was one of his goats. He never places his hand on Freddy. Half of me feels happy about this. The other half is very angry. Jealous even.

'Mother what does amputation mean?' She screams and hacks the chicken carcass, punctuating each word. 'You selfish pig! I feed you an extra bowl of rice for the sake of your brother. You think he likes being carried by somebody who wants to chop him into tiny bits?' Chop, chop, chop. Chicken pieces fly in every direction, till there is nothing left. She collects the small parts and with another smart slap tells me to get away from her or I will soon regret it.

The wind whistles in all directions on the rocky outcrop above our home. Here clouds pass by to rain on the villages below. My angry tears are collected by them and I cheer up since Mother cannot stop me from imagining Freddy stretched out on a gleaming surgical bench, a necrotic remnant of me. I imagine him being placed in a jar of formaldehyde for me to admire like a souvenir when I have nothing better to do. It is my one consolation as I rub the red spot on my cheek and return to the hut.

Each night Mother bathes us in olive oil. It is a ritualistic practice that I have always accepted without question. She sings under her breath while I inhale the labour of her day, her armpits passing over my face. She prays in the dim, taper lit hut. She hurries over me, with her there, there care and then takes her time to caress Freddy carefully, gently. Her weathered features soften and her breathing slows as if she has found peace through placing her hands upon Freddy. My Father rocks in his chair, lost in the depths of the fire while she massages my brother in small circular motions. She blesses his soul and offers up thanks while holding one finger across my sealed lips. She kisses me and tells me I must rise early to help my brother prepare for the journey to town tomorrow. I watch her retreat from my small wooden cot.

Alone, Freddy laughs his head off. Inside my ribs hurt as if something hard is pushing them apart. He does it every night after he is bathed and blessed. I can feel my body jiggle with his joy. With Mother gone, I slap his bottom hard. 'It isn't funny.' More chortling and my stomach churns full of mixed emotions, half digested food and unanswered questions. 'I hate you!' Freddy stops. I would reject him but it isn't me who has the choice. He is the other son my Mother loves while I wish he was nothing more than an appendage. Only half of me can truly love him. He is the one who is not fully formed but my Mother feels he makes up for this by trumping me with his silent wisdom. I smack him again. After all, it won't hurt me. I turn my body toward the hut wall, cupping Freddy carefully as I make myself comfortable. I move his hand from under me so it won't get squashed. 'Thank you' echoes through me. I sniff and reply gruffly 'It's nothing.' We lie there. I feel the odd one out. How can I ever be complete with something half-finished attached to me? Freddy shakes his head inside of me. 'You're a good brother. I shouldn't laugh at you but I think it is because I love you.' I would turn my back on him but it just isn't possible. 'How would I know happiness without you?' Freddy's love flows through my veins and I feel his body glow as we share this mutual moment. He needs me. Perhaps I need him. I kiss my hand and rub his slippery back. Eventually I burp and we both settle down for the night.

Hydra: A Poem for People With Voices in their Heads (4rensicDJ)

Hydra with your seven heads,
Tormenting me with things I dread,
Speaking to me so sour,
I cannot take this another hour.
Debilitating my personality,
The suffering I feel is a calamity.
Do with me what you will,
Because this cannot be fixed with some little pill.
You have been around since before I remember,
Since the very first December,
And I still remember that day,
And how you tormented me in such a way,
But I am used to you now,
However your torment remains anyhow.
When you let up?
When will I say enough is enough?
Why can't I stay away?
Maybe because this pain is part of my day to day.

Visiting Hour (MissingLink)

While you work out the algorithms
of a single weed
pushing its way through
the cracked concrete,
I will stretch my arms
around you
till I can tie them in a bow.
We can rattle off,
I'd like to teach the world
to sing
in perfect harmony
Perhaps,
just perhaps
the rest of the garden
will waken
from its catatonic state.

The Light Inside the Shadow

Trapped—A Story about Mental Illness (4rensicDJ)

She was lost and trapped. Not trapped in a physical sense, but she was trapped in the world, and within herself. And that has always been the worst kind of trapped; to feel trapped within yourself feels like you have no options, nowhere to go, no means of living.

She ran through the forest, her feet cut and bruised, her hair strewn across her face, stuck to her forehead with sweat and mud. She was running from something, to somewhere; but she didn't know from what, or where she was headed. She ran for the sake of running, she was trying to get away from this physicality that was following her, but all she really wanted to do was get away from herself. That was something impossible, so she ran.

The cold night created goose bumps up her arm, and it felt as though the cold was soaking through her skin to her innards, chilling her whole system, making any movement send a shooting pain through her limbs. But she didn't mind, she had felt worse pain. She extended her arms to push branches from her path, but it did more detriment than it helped. The branches were sharp and made wounds in her hands and the branches didn't move out of her way. She cried loudly in exasperation and pain, but she figured at least her hands were warmed by the sticky liquid.

What was ahead for her? What pain would she meet once she got to where she was going? Because there was always pain that followed and tormented her. When one pain left, another one returned in its place, sometimes a new foe but more often than not it was an old one. Would anyone help her? These questions would only be answered when she stopped running, and she knew that; but could she ever stop? This she did not know.

Further and further into the forest she ran. At least she believed she was going deeper, when in actually fact she was on the brink of breaking through the line of trees. She tripped and fell, scraping her chin on the roots of the forest floor. She stayed lain there for minutes, maybe even hours, crying into the ground; she had forgotten all about running. She was breaking.

She felt a hand on her back which forced her to open her eyes quickly. She sat up and pushed her way back into a tree. She didn't trust anyone, she was afraid of contact; she knew they brought more pain. She looked up to meet her maker, but the face she was confronted with was soft and kind. The slightly tanned face was framed by long light brown hair, flowing in waves to her ribs, with fringe pinned to the side with a feather that looked like one a gypsy would wear. The woman smiled at her, showing off her dimples and lighting up her eyes. She was still wary, but she got to her feet slowly, still cautious, merely to look in the woman's eyes. They were shining and had oranges, gold, greens and browns swimming in them. She could see the pain in them, even though she knew the woman was trying to hide it. She could see the pain that mirrored her own; this woman had seen pains one should not see, in some ways more pain than she herself had seen. This pain- these eyes- are what forced her to trust this woman, so that when the woman extended her hand, she gingerly laid her hand within it and allowed the woman to lead her out of the forest. It was such pain that enabled her to reply when the woman whispered tenderly, 'My name's Deej,' she replied softly, her voice cracking momentarily, 'I'm Fi.'

Her new friend, 'Deej', once out of the forest, led her to a huge tent, one like she had never seen before. It stood at least five times taller than her and was red and white striped with lots of colourful flags around it, decorating what was holding it into the ground. She was a little intimidated by the massive structure; where she came from there was nothing like this. Where she came from. The thought of where she had left sent a long shiver down her back. She hated it and never wanted to go back to such a horrific place. Deej sensed a feeling of sadness and hesitation in her companion, so she placed a comforting arm around her and slowed her walk.

"It's okay, this is one of the friendliest places on Earth," Deej whispered. Fi looked up at Deej and searched her colourful eyes for lies and deceit, but was only met with kindness and honesty. She even managed a slight smile to match the beaming the one on Deej's warm face.

They eventually reached the front of the tent structure and as Deej pulled back the flap to the entrance, Fi gasped slightly and cowered behind Deej. The tent opened up into a wide space, with plastic seating surrounding a central circle, which had about a dozen people on it. Deej reassured her companion of the safeness and love in the place and helped her come forward. The people in the circle all stopped what they were doing and came to look at the new girl. They examined her, looking up and down, tutting and shaking their heads. Fi whimpered and grasped Deej's arm. This was just like her home; people judging her. Fi felt stupid for assuming this place would be any different.

She looked around at all the people, some had juggling balls in their hands, others had strange make-up smothered on their face, some stood feet over Fi's height, and many of the girls had pretty dresses on with jewels and gorgeous white legs. Fi admired them all individually, taking the time to fully process the beauty she saw. They all smiled and nodded at her, instead of shaking their heads like before. She could sense the respect they all had for Deej. Fi looked up at Deej as a small child looks up at a parent.

"This is the Blue Circus, home of all strange outcasts. This is where you'll finally fit in." Fi still looked unsure about joining this band of misfits, but something made her walk forward. Perhaps it was the strength she felt emanating from Deej or the safeness of Deej as well, or could it be she was just happy to be inside for once? Whatever it was, it made her feel as though she was finally home.

During the next few days, Fi never left Deej's side. There was something about Deej that made Fi stay with her, that made Fi trust her. Deej showed her around the tent and introduced her to the animals. Fi's favourite people, save Deej, were ones named Si, Pirate and Peggy. Si was an amazing juggler and Fi would sit with Deej and watch him juggle for hours. Pirate was a weight lifter, and Peggy was a contortionist. In her own strange way, Fi began to admire them all, began to look at them as if they were her own family; look at Deej as if they were long lost twins. The only time Fi and Deej were not together was at night time, and even then Fi felt connected to the mesmerising Deej in a powerful way. Fi would often awaken from her slumber to sharp pains in her chest, before hearing screams come from Deej's trailer. Whenever Fi heard this she was pained, and hearing Deej in such pain hurt like Fi never thought she could be hurt; she now knew where one source of that intricate pain that layered Deej's eyes came from, a beast that attacked her at night. In the mornings, Deej would always appear from her trailer with scabs and scars, but the smile never left her face; Deej would be strong for Fi, because Fi was everything to Deej.

Fi often found herself observing Deej, from afar, and every now and then, she would attempt to sketch her as she worked. Fi was not that good of a drawer, but she had a particular style that seemed to suit Deej's being, so she drew. Fi always drew Deej laughing, but the pain in her eyes were always captured. The reason Fi could draw such pain in such beautiful eyes? She drew her own, but added many more layers of hurt.

Fi eventually mustered up the courage one night to ask Deej what beast tortured her at night. Deej looked at Fi, a smile spread across her face as she whispered 'Nothing but that which I deserve' before retiring for the night. It angered Fi in a strange way to hear Deej say she deserved such a horrible presence in her life, and Fi's opinion of Deej warped slightly.

Truth changes a person, and to hear Deej's version of the truth made Fi momentarily question if Deej really did deserve such a thing. She knew in her heart that it was not true, but when do people really listen solely to their hearts without letting their heads impact? Rarely. Fi started to go off on her own, letting Pirate teach her weightlifting techniques and Peggy help her become more flexible. Fi started taking care of the animals as well, a job that was meant for Deej.

However Deej did not mind; her beautiful friend, Fi, was finally fitting in, finally had a place she could truly call home. Deej stood against a pole and watched Fi laugh with Peggy as they fed the monkeys, when Si came up beside her and threw a loving arm around her shoulders.

'She is a good kid, you chose well,' He whispered.

Deej smiled to herself. 'I did not choose her, she came to us by some miracle and it was merely my duty to help her along the way. But there is a darkness and a light that follow her, there was something chasing her in the woods when I found her. The light within her consists of darkness and it is only a matter of time before it follows her here.'

Deej stated all of this to Si in rather a blunt manner. Deej knew as Fi did; you should distance yourself from getting personally attached, it merely brought hurt. But there was something about this beauty, about this girl who seemed younger than Deej but was obviously older, that made Deej want to be attached. She saw herself in Fi, as Fi saw herself in Deej.

Si looked at Deej worried. 'Deej, we are not warriors.'

'No, we are not. But for her-for family-we will always fight.' And with that, Deej walked back to her trailer and did not emerge for days...

The Light Inside the Shadow

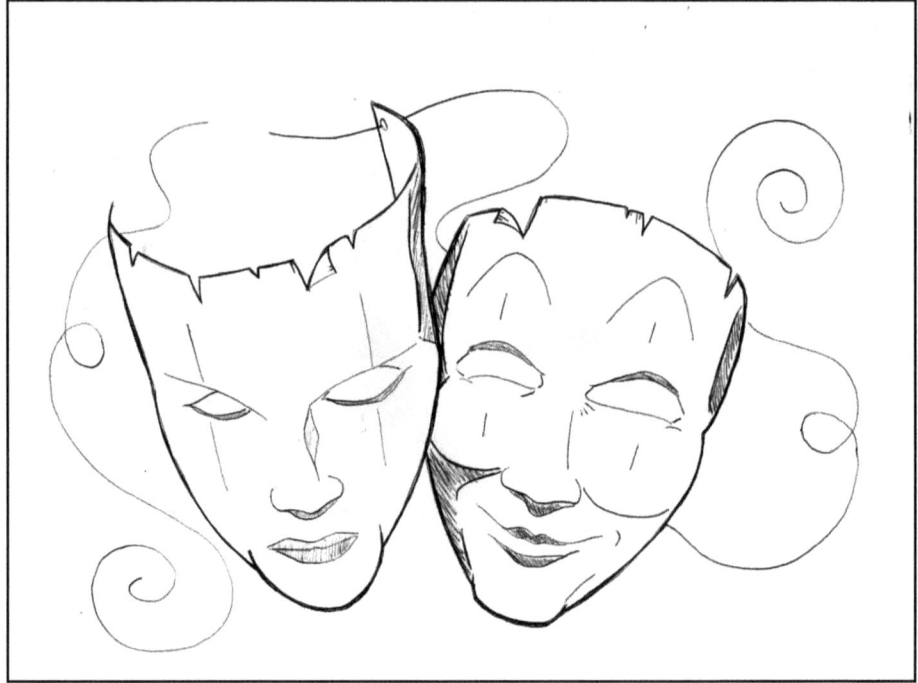

My Curse (GonePirate)

Rats (MissingLink)

My pantry door is wide open.
Come, weave between
the tins of damaged kidney beans,
a baby's silk shoe in the flour bin
and the crumbs of auntie's
special fruit cake from a christmas
I was too pissed to remember.

Bottles of half finished
sauces,
congealed drizzles at the nozzles,
a reminder that chips in newspaper
were a crime against humanity.
While I nested expectantly,
your photograph was pasted
on the inside of the door
next to the grubby measurements
of some unknown child
cast out into the world,
snared by her insatiable greed.

All this happened
long before I made footprints in the turmeric,
long before my rodent droppings
mattered

The Light Inside the Shadow

The Dog (4rensicDJ)

My deepest, darkest fears,
Being brought to light.
The horrible words;
My inability to fight.
The mean memories,
And shattering heart break;
I need to keep fighting,
But I can't for God's sake!
The voices in my head,
All shout negativities at me.
I need to let go;
I want to be free.
But I cannot,
And so here they remain.
They whisper 'You're not good enough';
And other terrible things that cause me great pain.
So here I am,
With these thoughts in my head.
I wish to get them out,
But I can't, I dread.

What This Does (4rensicDJ)

As I stood there, staring into his cold brown eyes, I could see all the years of lies flashing in them, the demons that he never exorcized threatening to break through. They seemed to play within his eyes; they seemed to laugh at the water slowly building on his lower eyelid. My face dropped as I knew there was little I could do to save him.

I saw tear drops hit the ground and without looking up, I embraced him, trying to pass my warmth, trying to pass the small morsel of happiness that still existed within me, to him. Hearing him sob softly into my shoulder made tears form in my own eyes and I patted his back feeling so helpless, I couldn't do anything else.

So many thoughts raced through my head; what made him break like this, so suddenly? How did I show him things were going to be alright? What was I ever going to do to try and make this pain easier, to try and convince him to stay with me? The last question sent a shiver down my spine. If he left, if I had to survive without him, I wouldn't last long, I would be so completely lost I wouldn't be able to function, let alone live.

"Bub," I whispered, clutching him tightly, so afraid to let go. "Bub, sweetie, you gotta talk to me, I have to try and help you." He gripped me harder, I could feel his fingers digging into my skin and his sobs got heavier. I could feel him shaking his head in my shoulder and my face creased heavily, trying to hold back the tears that were threatening to spill over and make things worse.

After several moments of silence besides the constant sobbing emanating from him, he pulled out of my hug. I clutched his back, I tried to keep him against me, keep him close and keep him safe, but he pulled my hands off him, holding them and looking into my eyes as I did his. I hated that he wasn't as close to me as I wanted, but I bared it for his sanity rather than mine.

His face was red and streaked from the tears, his nose running and his eyes puffy. He tilted his head slightly with a small pout, and I knew he was trying to fight back more tears.

"Sweetie, please," I pleaded, pulling his hands to my chest and holding them there, looking into his eyes and begging silently for him to let me in. His face fell as he frowned heavily and his tears began again. And now my own tears started. I didn't want them to, I was trying to hold it in, for him, to be strong because he needed me to be strong right now, but I couldn't anymore. Not after seeing him like that, it was too much, and it broke my heart like I never thought it could be broken.

I embraced him again, and although I couldn't hear him crying, I could feel my jumper becoming more wet with his tears. He had reached his numb crying stage and that scared me even more. My tears came down harder as I clutched to him, this time making sure not to let go.

"I ****ed up Deej," He stated monotonously. I gripped him tighter, burying into his shoulder and shaking my head. "I did Deej, I screwed up really bad and I failed you; I failed myself."

I kept my head buried in the nook between his neck and his shoulder, not wanting to move, trying to figure out a way to show him how much I cared, how much I wanted to help and how I'd never leave, no matter what he did.

"You didn't, you didn't bub," I whispered, the words muffled and momentarily lost in the fabric of his hoodie. I could feel his head nod and I couldn't help myself, I pulled back and kissed him on the cheek, my lips becoming salty from the remnants of his tears.

When I pulled back, he looked stunned and I couldn't tell if he was happier or not; he just stared at me blankly. I clutched his hands in mine again; scared he'd run and leave, and looked at him with sorrow in my eyes. It didn't even matter what he thought he'd done wrong; it never mattered how hard he'd betrayed my trust. I would stand by his side forever.

Tears filled my eyes and I stared at him, trying to make him see my love for him and I wasn't sure he could.

"I... I," I stumbled, trying to grab words but they just kept evading my capture. I tried desperately to think of something to say that would make him feel better. "I don't know how I can help. But I want to," I managed to get out. I couldn't see his reaction to my statement through my tears, his whole being was blurry; but I knew he had retaken my hands in his, clutching them so tightly I could feel the bones rubbing against each other.

"I'm sorry," He whispered, his voice cracking with pain. The pain within his voice hit me like a brick wall and made every emotion I was feeling much more real and agonizing.

"You promised you'd stay with me," My voice had now begun to shake along with my hands, my breathing becoming sporadic and my thoughts racing faster than I thought humanly possible.

"I know, I told you I failed you." I felt his hands slip out of mine, I wiped my tears and I saw him start to walk away. I ran after him, pulled him back around to face me and hugged him so tightly there was no air between our bodies. He embraced me too, wrapping his arms around me with his hands at the small of my back.

"You could never fail me," I whispered into his ear, my face crinkled in anguish. "I'm proud you're still here."

He didn't say anything in return. There was no more space for our bodies to get any closer but somehow my grip tightened and I managed to close the non-existent gap.

"You give me hope," I murmured. I felt his arms tighten around my waist and I could feel his dimple against my cheek; the dimple that only came out when he was smiling.

Author's Note:

I wrote this story one day after coming home from a truly terrible day at school. What I've depicted in my story was not a true event, but was based around feelings I knew other people had towards me. So I decided to write a story from my perspective as if I was one of my friends that was having to deal with my depression and anxiety and all other mental illnesses and how I knew it affected them.

What I hope this story does is shed some light on mental illness, that it doesn't only affect the person who has been diagnosed with it; it also takes a toll on those who care about you. Now, this is not something to feel guilty for, something to be simply aware of. People who are very dear to me have snapped at me before, and previously I thought it was all my fault, but I soon realised that my depression was taking an emotional toll on them and if anything, I shouldn't hold them in a higher light to myself, I should treat them like someone exactly like myself because if anything they were experiencing this themselves via proxy.

I ramble somewhat, I apologise; my message is simply this. Don't get too mad at yourself or those around you, if they (or even you) distance themselves (yourself) for a period of time before returning. They still love you and care about you, and if you're distancing yourself you know it's out of love, they just need some time to get themselves back together emotionally so they can continue to help you. If they run themselves dry and don't heal, they could end up one of us, and as much as I have come to accept my mental illnesses; I wouldn't wish them on anyone.

Living in the World

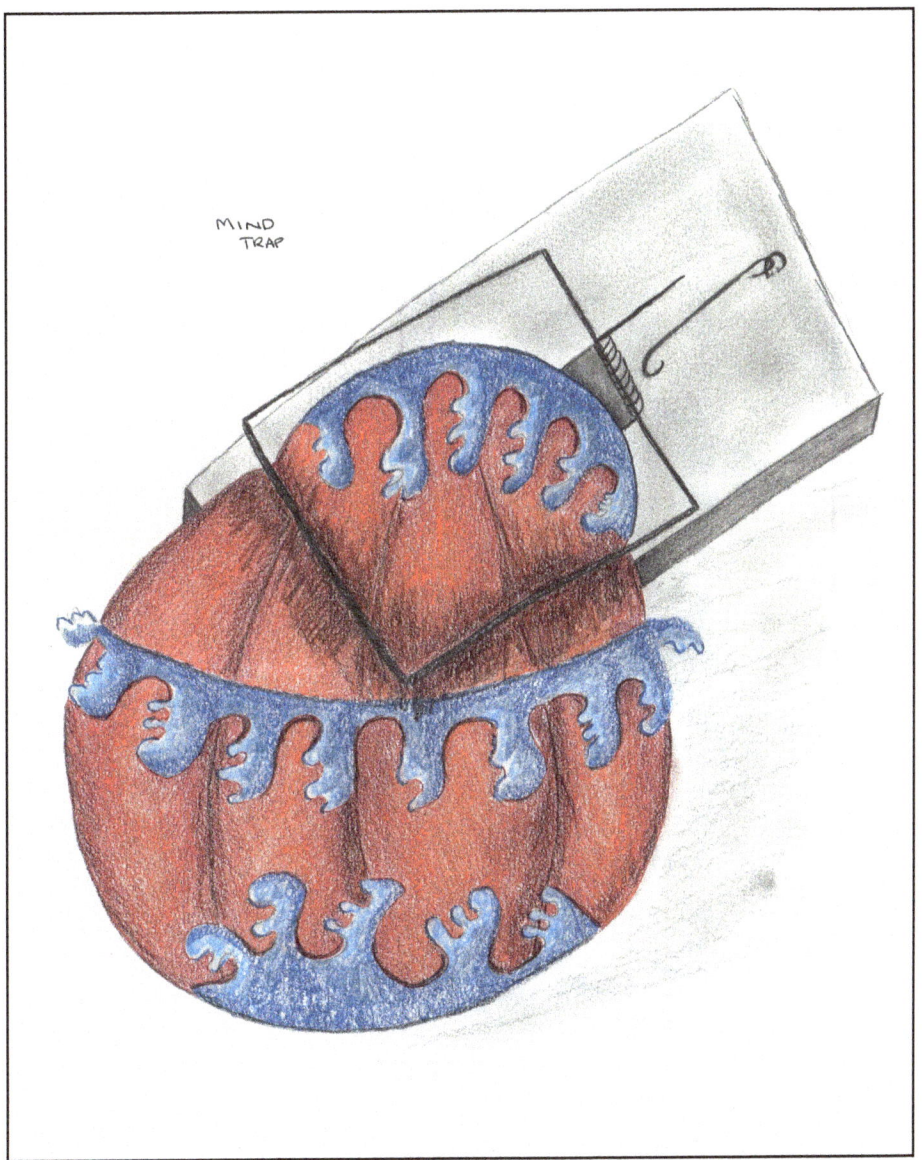

Mind Trap (snowy)

Even in the few weeks that come occasionally, when I am stable, my whole being is still trapped by the demands of this disease. They said "anything is possible" when I was growing up – they lied.

The Light Inside the Shadow

Without Hesitation (creative)

Without hesitation
I walked away
for I knew I would not win
for I knew there was no reasoning
the system wins
so we live without wisdom
so we live without peace
this is our life.

So many times I've asked myself
where's the hope in all of that?
seems to me we are just fumbling
in a verbosity
in false understandings
in misguided truths
that lead us nowhere.

If I could show you the world I live in
then you would join me in an instant
then you would see the simple truth
you would feel the love inside
love that keeps you warm.

And then I knew there was no chance
you would ever come my way
you would never dare to look
for the truth always hurts
you rather dismiss me
pretend I am not there
to protect your conscience

But the truth always finds you
it will stay there in your heart
and you tell me that you know
but that life is what it is
seasons come and seasons go.

My whole philosophy in life is this (GonePirate)

my whole philosophy in life is this
this is my life, and life is a collection of moments,
don't spend those moments making memories you'd rather forget,
instead try pursue happiness with a little diligence,
but a conclusion I believe I have found is this.
that as a society humans ain't worth shit
the things they do that demolish their dignity
their lack of self respect really saddens me
a frivolous, trivial, arrogant mob,
egocentric, ignorant , arrogant slobs
the majority of which disgustingly,
seems to make no sense to me,
respect in one's self isn't asking too much
but faith in mankind is lost among us,
perhaps a conclusion is I just don't like people
but surely this dilemma cannot be that simple
with no humanity in an inhuman world
where all your depravities will come unfurled
hate is a strong word I do believe so
only a few in this world truly know
even those rare have seldom embraced it
taken the hate in your grasp and just taste it
man is remarkably selfish and needy as hell
malicious and mean and greedy as well
this tortured reality is slightly broken
as my long distant words are so faintly spoken
is there hope for mankind left after sorrow
there is no way to see when there is no tomorrow
so never give in because times are a rough
no one ever survived a battle without skin that's tough
and life is just that a challenge a war
it can make you, and shape you, and break you or more
anyone who survives is a hero indeed
anyone who cannot is a soul in dear need

The Light Inside the Shadow

the wanderer (GonePirate)

see the hatred in your eyes
I've paid the price, I've paid the cost
and now I've come to realise
not all who wander are lost...

we fade from vision (Miseries Company)

we fade from vision as we fade from thought, the heart has no memory for the broken soul, we become the ethereal we reach for the ground from deep below, we find our place in darkness, we feel not the pain of loss, cause we can no longer lose we can fall no further.

the mind aches as the heart breaks for all the loves never felt for all the friends that are never met, we feel our form dissipating becoming nothingness, we do not do anything to harm our self or others as that would be a breach of what holds us, we just fade away no one notices no one cares it's ok it has always been this way.

it is pain, it is hurt, it is me, to be strong, smart, quick witted, helpful, I could take people from the brink of this this me I could reform them, I could give them power back, maybe I was giving what I was, my power, I dont know, but in the end I was the one facing down the firing squad while they walked away without a care, I did not scream out, I did not beg, I faced it down, but in the end how many times can you face down that firing squad before the weight of lead drags you down, put my heart on the line for love just to watch the blade fall in the very hands of the person it would do anything for, there was many evils within my days yet I go on looking over that cliff, seeing the dark foreboding waves, not fearing them, but I will not cause hurt, I will not become that which I despise.

trust sadly it must be earned from me now, something that once was so easily given without fear, just cant be given anymore, and well if no-one felt the want to accept it when it was so easy to acquire, then surely no one will care now that it would need to be earned, but oh well, so be it, gotta deal I guess

would that it could show upon my skin the scars of many wounds inflicted to me in the name of love, my skin would no longer show, as it would be merely scars upon scars, the love of friends betrayed and destroyed by subversive thoughts and actions bought forth upon me by the very ones I trust with all my soul.

my love, desire and devotion to those I wished would return my love and would be mine as I would be theirs, wreaked naught but rejection and humiliation on me yet of course they would take from me what they wanted, my strength, my mind, while they reveled in their enjoyment at my ignorant and foolish heart as they enjoyed others with their heart and body, all the while laughing inside at the pathetic creature that would be there through all time to help them when they hurt, pick them up when they fall, fight in their name against the evils that would come for them, and love them all the while.

a heart that beats for all within my breast a seemingly strong exterior that shows no pain, a male form that is made and taught to never show its weaknesses stands firm, the tears that rip through my insides like waves crashing against a beach that shalt not fall except for in those very few times that my dam walls can no longer contain the force of the encroaching tide.

a heart that wishes beyond all that it could have one with which to beat its full force and have theirs beat a return chorus, yet can it be the mind yells "no" the heart screams "yes" which is right or are they both wrong, does that one exist or is that merely a dream meant to never come true, and if they were to exist how would one such as me know, a me that is now so weak, so fractured, can see so much yet is blind to the heart of others, maybe it just is not meant to be.

to all things there must come an end, my only dream, my only aspiration, my only true desire was to find love, to have a family, yet it seems this to must reach its end, if it is as it shall be then it is meant to never change.

oh cruel book of fate why was it enforced on me this strength to feel so strongly when it was not meant to be that I should see my feelings returned to me, it is the curse of me the heart of depth, the vision to see their pain, the power to help lessen their pain, yet for me it was never meant to be that I should feel another's heart, my heart beats for one and shall continue to till it's time to stop, will it ever know true love the outlook is bleak, will it ever feel another beating with it, the signs are not strong.

would that it could be that feelings could stop, sadly they cannot so my big heart breaks a little each day for a love it will never know, but with my heart I go on, everyone lets go but me, even if I walk away I never let go, because it is not meant to be that I should forget, I see the faces of those I have loved and cared for each still holds a piece of my heart, their images flash against my retinas and will until that dark day when it is lost this beautiful heart.

why is it we can never just be (GonePirate)

why is it we can never just be
are we children of the sea
this is the truth as spilt by me
a man who chases fate endlessly
pulled by tides and pushed by waves
finding cold and wet watery graves
but I carry on with every passing sun
tirelessly preparing the ship until done
for the next voyage the next journey
of personal experience and self learning
we're lost children of the sea
we chase joy endlessly
into day and through the night
into combat, to battle and fight
through the weeks and into months
years of depravity down in dumps
through the years and into decades
chase the joy with tongues like blades
that cut the life out of lifeless foes
who stood for things that no one knows
but the reason we can never be
is we are born and drawn to the sea
born to chase joy endlessly
drawn to return unto the sea.

this small ship surrounding me
carries me to where I be
I am a man, who's lost at sea
Poseidon, what have you planned for me
the tides they come in and call to me
tirelessly and longingly
I am lost I'm lost at sea
Poseidon, what have you planned for me
the shore, the shore is blind to me
the sea, the seas are all that I can see
I am a man, a man lost at sea
Poseidon, what do you demand of me
blinded by sun shine upon the sea
blinded by fate drawn on endlessly
I am a man, a man lost at sea
Poseidon why must you keep chasing me

The Light Inside the Shadow

    is this my punishment, that's my only question
    to live in squalor, without any possessions
    to be a man so fueled by aggression
    a heartless pirate with no direction
    why is this my life? That's my query
    this pirate has only one theory
    but I cannot manage to speak clearly
    so I turned to the seas and held them dearly
    but the persona of a sane man that I'm using
    I hold on to tightly but I find I'm losing
    the battle with my demons is an illusion
    I'm circling the ocean, a delusion
    when truth grips me the force is bruising
    a scoundrel used to live for boozing
    living his life by his own choosing
    on the sea with crew just cruising

    but with this ship surrounding me
    that carries me to where I be
    I am a man, who's found the sea
    Poseidon, do your worst to me
    the tides they come in and call to me
    tirelessly and longingly
    I am found I'm found at sea
    Poseidon, just try stopping me
    the shore, the shore is blind to me
    the sea, the seas are all that I can see
    I am a man, a man who knows the sea
    Poseidon please stop tempting me
    blinded by sun shine upon the sea
    blinded by fate drawn on endlessly
    I am a man, a man lost at sea
    Poseidon why must you haunt me

    as winds shift and waves roll on and on.
    a ship cutting sea endlessly towards freedom
    sail off into the sunset to find yourself in the black
    but to have come so far there's no turning back
    an' after all the seas these long years I've crossed
    and with every race to the horizon I've seen lost
    I still chase that feeling like the nights chase day
    my compass is true but still guides me away,
    I long for the taste of something free

something born inside of me
something that's drawing me closer to the sea.
that is where I need to be
we are the masters of our own demise
as the torrent seas surround us rise
lost in the seas of truth
long since wasted away my youth
now homesick for a place I've never been.
and far more familiar with sights I've never seen.
do we hold the world in our grasp, do we hold life in our hands.
take to the guiding wind just as the sea commands
throw your anchors away they hold you back and bring you down.
cast away your sails as the winds will turn you 'round
as our bellies cry for a beggar's feed we find ourselves broke
and in our desperation we breathe fire and smoke
with stomachs full of tar and oil we all roared and cried
and pillaged all around us until the whole world died
in confusion we seek death to feel alive
and in our delusion we find it hard to survive.
but my fortitude is strong and by my siren's song
this pirate's been sailing so long, singing this tired old song
with a yo and a ho I think its time for home
only to find the seas I've seen are the only home I've known

The Light Inside the Shadow

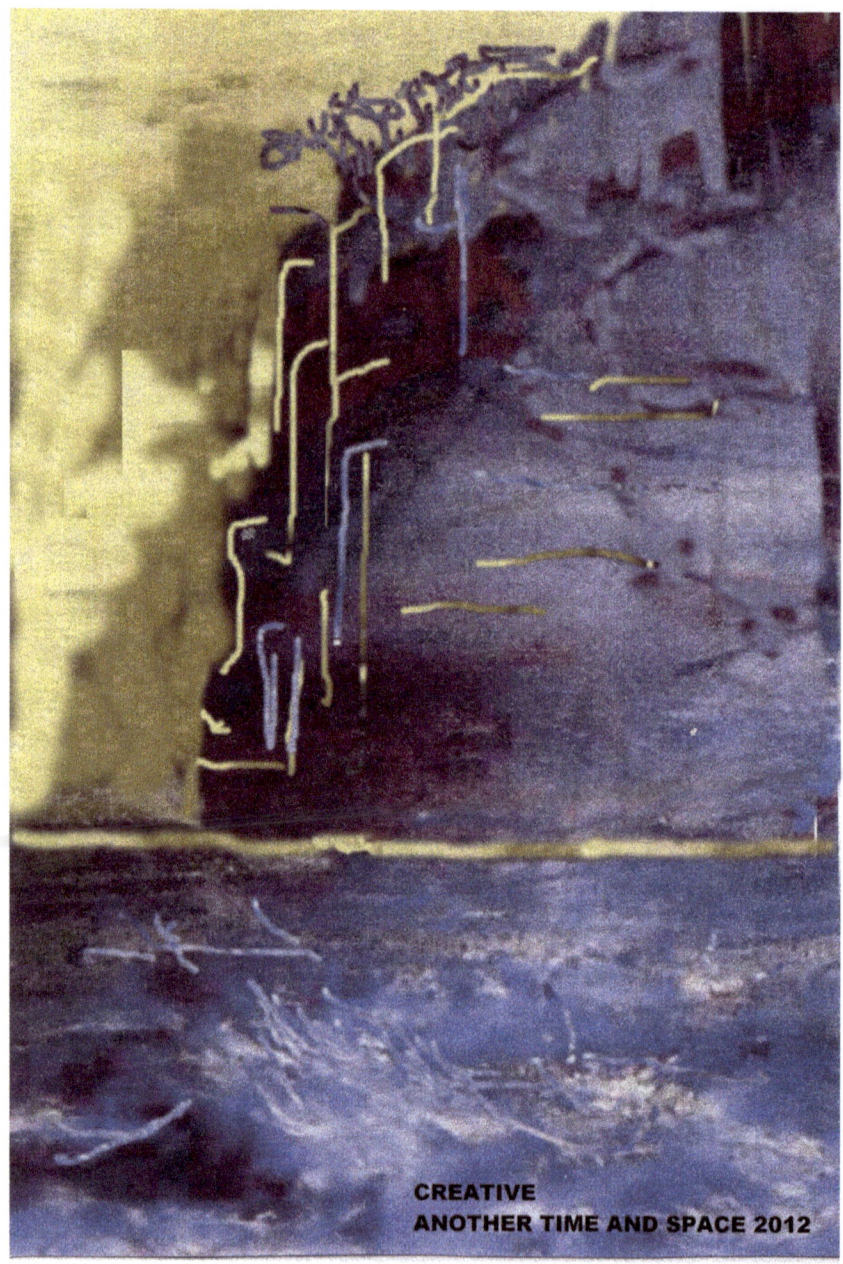

Another Time and Space (creative)

This painting was partly inspired by my synesthesia and the title "Another time and space" indicates my impression, or fantasy, of having lived in another space and time: a much better, more complete existence than my current one.

Paddling Back (MissingLink)

Up above the noisy traffic,
the intersection,
the honking noise,
it's difficult to row back
without going round
in circles.
My umbrella oars
pop open,
as if their close proximity
to the clouds tell them,
'here it gets stormy'
My wishes won't navigate me safely
to where I want to be.
Me wearing my favourite bikini
with feet no bigger than a child's.
But umbrella oars never paddle
fast enough.
Not enough to escape bad memory rips
that suck you in for all eternity.
Here I wish for SOS patterns in the sky,
hoping I can avoid a crash landing.
My feet are just too small now
to walk the long distance home.

The Light Inside the Shadow

When I was a child (stressbunny)

I never would have dreamed when I was only young
that storm clouds would move in and take away the sun,
that joy would fall from my clear blue sky
and dark shadows would come sailing by.

I never would have dreamed that when I got older
worry would hurt me like a wounded soldier,
it would taunt me, tease me and tip me over
until I had simply lost all composure.

I never would have dreamed when I was a little girl
when everything was beautiful and precious like a pearl,
that my mental health would break
and my heart forever ache.

I never would have dreamed that God would not listen
when I prayed for His help none came to my prison,
I was locked in my anguish and locked in my pain
depression had beat me and anxiety had gained.

I never would have dreamed that my mind would be my foe
that thoughts would panic me or make me really low,
and friends would slowly back away
because they knew not what to say.

I never would have dreamed that my family wouldn't care
instead they stood in pride for fear of despair,
a mental illness is not acceptable to them
must I suffer in silence so not to offend?

I never would have dreamed that dreams may never be
that prayers go unanswered and I can't be free,
so now I dream I was just a child once more
when only peace and joy came to my front door

Absent Father (MissingLink)

Sitting on your lap
safe from the world
Whiskers rubbing
against my cheek
while I brushed your sideburns
and I'll never forget
the smell of blue stratos
mingled with cigarettes
while I nestled there
as you finished
your last pint
Years later
I saw these threads
felt them
as your hand went
limp
then your eyes closed
after gazing at me
in your final moment
at what seemed like
a lifetime
captured in a few small
seconds
You breathed out
I breathed in
at the wonder of it all
thinking I was a gift to you
that you never unwrapped
I wonder what you
ever were to me.

The Light Inside the Shadow

I miss you (GonePirate)

do you think about me now and then
will we ever be together again
I close my eyes and see you in a vision
I want to have you again it's my decision
but want is a two person dance
but all I ask for is a second chance
I'd do anything to make you smile
even though I haven't seen you in a while…
you're still the one for me, the only one I need
the only one for whom I'd tear my heart out and bleed
you can illuminate me with just a look
and I can read your face like an open book
I miss you more each day, as you're out there free
flying around without a thought for old me
but I was the first who ever saw something in you
I was the first to love you it's true
I was the first to break your heart
I was the one from the very start
but I couldn't handle it I had to go
for reasons that I finally understand and know
I was sick and you were in pain
I made you go completely insane
acting in a way that just wasn't meant to be
you just started acting, acting like me…
if I could undo this I surely would
if I could renew this I surely should
because living without you in my life
is like living a husband without his wife
I want you I need you I love you as well
and without your light my life is just hell.

The Light Inside

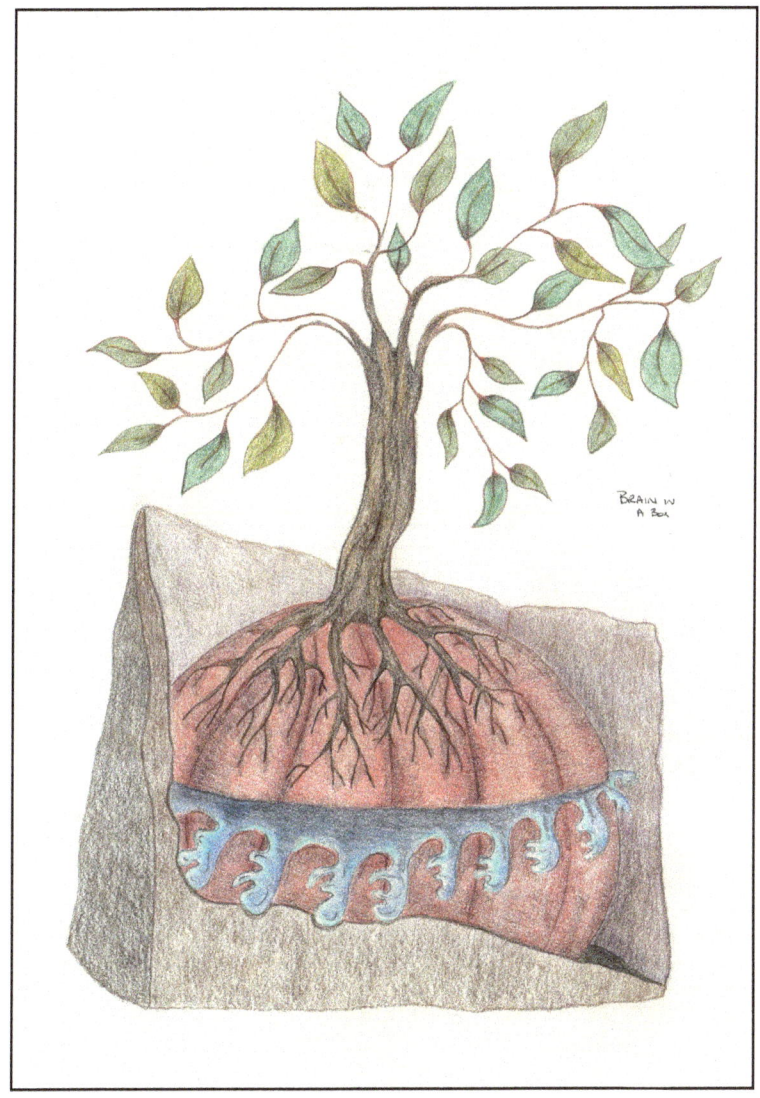

Brain in a Box (snowy)

This is from a time I felt so ill, damaged and worn out that I could no longer care what happened to me. It just didn't matter anymore if I lived or died. When asked what would help, I wanted someone to put my brain in a box and look after it until it was well. I couldn't do it anymore and was so willing to destroy it all. The tree represents strength, the strength I desperately needed then and the strength I need on a daily basis to cope with this disease. This feeling happens often.

The Light Inside the Shadow

Baby Squeigh (Squeigh)

From adverse circumstances one can be born,
A Pegasus, the flying cloud child comes forth,
Pristine and white, pure and of hope,

The little Pegasus continues to grow. Through broken wings and bruised bones the Pegasus still continues to grow. No matter the pain, her heart is the core and violent flame.

Through all that the Pegasus endures it allows her to find the truth inside her soul. Those who never see themselves miss the truth the Pegasus sees, for one can not forever flee thyself. Strength in confronting who you are and allowing others to see your scars, to bare your soul and let them see who you really can be.

The Pegasus flies and will always try to fly, She sees the beacon of hope that remains alive. And if she can she is willing to take you on her back and fly you too.

I am the victim (Newleaf)

I am the victim
but also the bully

I am the rescuer
but also the one who chose to run away.

I am the outraged listener
But also the sympathetic reader.

I am the traitorous friend
But also the loyal ally.

We are a family
We are connected
We are one
Forgiveness is possible
Forgiveness is possible.

The Light Inside the Shadow

Failure (TheBeautifulBlueButterfly)

We can get art out of failure
Lessons out of failure
Hope out of darkness and despair
The light may be hiding under hundreds of layers
But no matter what, it's still there

"So what?" Says the failure
"I don't want to know."
I suppose like most failures, he lost hold of the railings and now he's content in that hole on his own
But there is life in that failure
Still a chance for that failure
To find the right path home

Today brings a poem of cheerful news
However I've been a failure too
And if I'm realistic I'll admit
I will see myself failing again before my life is through

We can find truth out of failure
Grow wiser out of failure
Even help the next failure through

Because we are all failures
That's how nature made us
Failure is not out to get you

The Taste Of Life (Silenus)

I have tasted life and now I humbly attempt to describe it,
All at once a food critic and evolving gourmand:
Three courses.

The entree was nice,
But I wasn't always mature enough to truly appreciate its simple splendour
(Though now I think back and remember the taste with fondness).

The main is delightfully complex, and,
Though not always pleasing to my palate,
It is the most wonderful course I have ever eaten.

The dessert I have yet to sample,
But from where I am sitting,
It looks absolutely delicious.

The accompanying drink is a rich and dry red,
At first fruity, but with a long peppery finish.
The glass appears always to be half full,
No matter how many draughts I take of it.
I even tipped the glass over once,
Clumsy and afraid,
And though it spilled onto the tablecloth,
When I righted it, it was as full as before.

Alas, the girl I was dining with has left,
But the empty chair across from me will not always be so,
For a meal shared tastes all the better...

The Light Inside the Shadow

Middle Age (MissingLink)

I've bashed corners
into circles
with each sweep
of life's broom.

Uncovered the mysteries
of dust balls
in dark, unused rooms.

So laugh with me
while I wash dishes;

before the bubbles
in the sink disappear.

The Light Inside

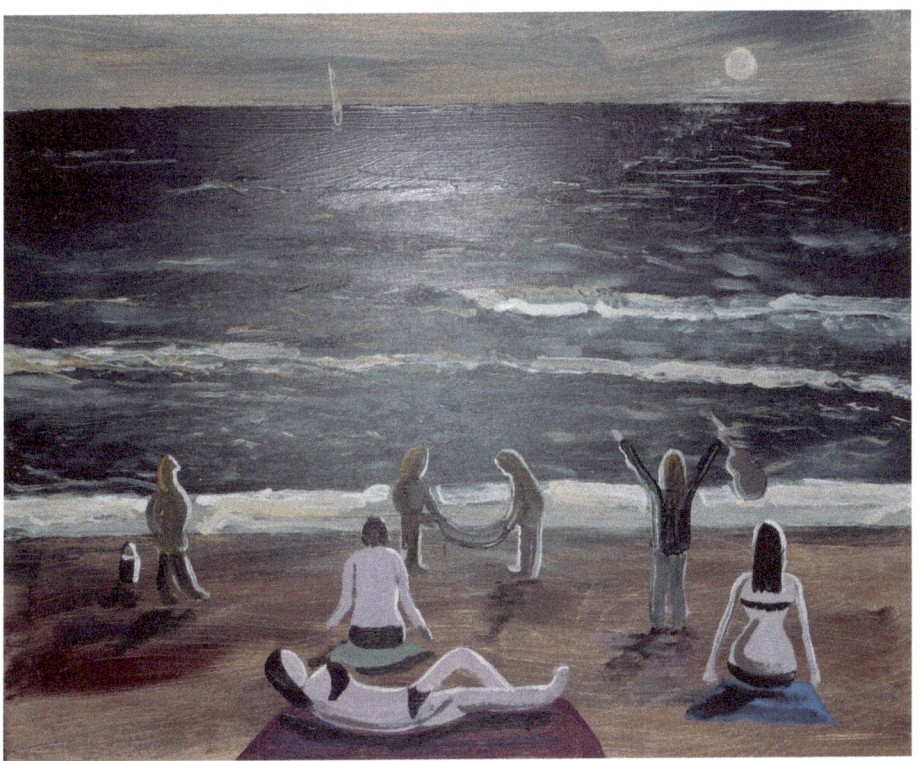

Moonbathers (creative)

Nowhere to hide (creative)

We are the forgotten people
with nowhere to hide;
we're dreamers of dreams
on whom the pale moon shimmers.

We transform the world;
being one with dreams,
one with love
one with art.

Ages come and ages go,
this we know:
each age has a dream dying,
or one that is rising to birth.

We sit and watch each age with its dream
one that passes, one that emerges
as the pale moon shimmers on our forgotten faces.

You Were There – My Story (Overtheedge)

An account from a survivor of childhood abuse

> With out-stretched wings I took to flight,
> Reveling with each breath the gift of life,
> With childhood dreams in my sight,
> I explored sandcastles, nature, games and Christmas nights
> Bathing in the warmth of my father's light,
> I felt his love ravage the night,
> With silver moons and dreams in sight,
> In my innocence I felt delight
> I looked around the empty walls,
> I no longer found my father's form,
> I turned to her who gave me life,
> I found eyes of steel and a glistening knife,
> I looked at her with love and fright,
> Mummy, mummy, are you alright?
> With a lash of fury and whipping of the tongue,
> "You worthless fool" her words had stung,
> You will never be anybody and friends will run,
> I knew my nightmare had just begun
> With the bath water running in the far off room,
> I was wondering if love would find me any time soon,
> Only to feel the pressure of her hand whilst under water,
> I was gasping for air like a lamb to the slaughter,
> But mummy, mummy, I am your daughter
> Suddenly I felt oxygen reprieve,
> And caught a glimpse of my father's sleeve,
> Dangling down around my mother's neck,
> Holding her up leaving me a train wreck
> Shadows and voices of the night,
> Started to echo terror with sheer delight,
> "Leave me alone" screamed a wretched sight,
> Blackened eyes beamed forward hysterical laughter at my plight,
> Oh God, Oh God, where is the light?
> Anger swept through my pores and took its toll,
> I rebel at you life you ugly troll,
> Broken mind and fractured soul,
> You left in my heart a gaping hole
> Man after man, wrong after wrong,
> Shattered dreams and emptiness came along,
> I realized life was not a game and this could not go on,

Enough is enough – where do I belong?
Anxiety, depression and fear rule the night,
I am sick of these obstacles in my sight,
There must be a purpose, an answer; God you must be somewhere,
I turned around and you were there
I still struggle with heart a-bleeding,
But you fulfill me with everything I am needing,
You are my angel, my shining light,
In you now I find delight

Author Statement

Depicted in this poetic piece is my personal experience of childhood abuse. My aim in sharing my story is to shed some light on the abuse that can go on behind closed doors, in many different forms, and the pain and terror suffered by victims. I wish to remove the taboo on this subject with the intention of bringing awareness to one of the most common triggers of mental illness. With awareness comes knowledge. With knowledge comes understanding.

With this understanding, it is my hope to remove some of the stigma associated with mental disorders, replacing it with compassion and acceptance of sufferers. I wish to encourage through my writing greater support of the mentally ill in our communities across Australia and the world, with providing better research and strategies towards sound mental health programs. I sincerely wish to see no more of the mentally ill living on our streets through no fault of their own. Some never had a chance from the outset.

I also wish to express through my writing to all who suffer at any stage of their lives, mental disorders, that there can be a light at the end of the tunnel if one never gives up. Love is the key.

A true story (creative)

I was 15 years old and, like all young boys, I had no understanding of real danger. That day we were playing hide and seek but the dangerous thing about this was that we were crossing a main busy road of six lines, back and forth. This was in a busy city. Eventually, as I was crossing for the tenth time, without caring too much about the dangers, I got hit by a white Combi Van. The impact was so powerful that I was lifted in the air, as my friends recall, and traveled for about 20 meters landing in the middle of the main road in peak traffic. Fortunately, I was not hit a second time. But I was dead: my heart had stopped and I had multiple fractures.

I remember a big bang sound and immediately after a wonderful peace and calmness. I was walking on air and was approaching a white tunnel, the tunnel of light. I felt a great desire to walk into this tunnel and to go further and further in it.

As I got close to the end, where the light really intensified, I heard a powerful voice say: "it is not your time, you need to go back. You should not be here." But I did not want to go back I was really enjoying the wonderful feeling of being there. And the voice said again: "only when it is your time can you cross the tunnel and get to the other side. Until your time comes, no matter what happens to you, or what you do to yourself, you will be sent back, one way or another." Soon after that, I woke up in the hospital and felt tremendous pain. I never forgot that experience and the immense pleasure of being in that tunnel of light. The doctors were able to get a heartbeat again and so I was resuscitated.

Ever since then, I have had periods of spirituality and periods where I stopped believing in anything. Like many people, I have been searching for answer to the riddle of life for many years. The experience of the tunnel, however, has always been proof, to me, that there is something really big out there that we cannot understand. No matter how hard I have tried to dismiss this and to say to myself that it was just a side effect of the shock, it felt very real and very meaningful.

The Light Inside the Shadow

The Beautiful Blue Butterfly (TheBeautifulBlueButterfly)

They probably think that I am too over analytical
Too emotionally unstable with too much baggage
They probably think that I am too lazy
Too unmotivated
Too awkward and crazy

They probably think that I am too chaotic
Trying so hard to make order out of a field of mess
Or maybe they think that I am too simplistic
Only able to take on minimal stress

Maybe I'm taking up too much room
Maybe I'm taking up too much time
Maybe I'm taking up too much attention, affection
Maybe I'm self indulged and stealing the limelight

Maybe I don't contribute enough
I may be too vulnerable or even too tough
I may always think and never act
I may focus too much on the things I lack

(But...)
I am a beautiful, inspiring, bright blue butterfly
With silver on my wings from all the times I've caught your cries
Moving in and out of shadows and constantly changing with the tide
I just cannot condone destruction when precious time is slipping by

So please try not to call me lazy
Useless, crazy or weak
Each insult is a dagger
One wound for every mean word you speak
I may be unstable
That is just the way I am
Remember, "unstable" becomes "stable"
With just one helping hand

Joy Ride (4rensicDJ)

This poem is dedicated to all of the people who never thought that happiness could be achieved with a mental illness... I am here to tell you that it is not necessarily the case <3

> You want me to write a happy poem,
> But I don't know how to show 'em.
> I write things of depression,
> That's all I really know,
> But then you come along,
> And let your happiness show.
> I have to learn from you,
> You need to teach me how to be,
> Because the fact of the matter is I need you,
> And I really think that you need me.
> Now I've got a flow,
> And a smile on my face,
> I think I can keep writing this poem,
> And still keep my grace.
> You bring happiness into my day,
> With you I can let myself shine,
> You make me so much better,
> And it's great that you're all mine.
> You make me feel really special,
> You teach me that I'm good enough,
> You bring light into my life,
> And I now know I don't always have to be tough.
> You know how to cheer me up,
> And always make me smile,
> And that's a really nice feeling,
> That I haven't had in a while.
> To me you are perfection,
> And I need you by my side,
> I cannot even express my joy,
> That there's someone with me on this wild ride.
> So if you ever feel down,
> Please just remember,
> That you are ever so important to me,
> And you will be in my heart forever!

The Light Inside the Shadow

Notice me? (squarepeg)

i can be strong
Notice me
i can stumble and fall
Notice me
i can have wise words to share
Notice me
i can still need a supportive hand
Notice me
i can stand independently
Notice me
i can feel lost and so alone
Notice me
i can climb veritable mountains
Notice me
i can feel so tired and weary
Notice me
i can think positively
Notice me
i can drown in thoughts of despair
Notice me
i can be here
Notice me
i can feel invisible
Notice me!

To those who watch on (stressbunny)

I've learnt a lot through suffering
and have simple advice
to those who watch on
at my gradual demise

I would simply say
straight from my heart
that to ask the right question
is where you must start

I'm not looking for answers
I'm not looking for help
From you I just want
a small question heart felt

Herein lies the answer
can you do this for me?
Just ask me this question
and we'll both feel free

"WHAT CAN I DO TO SUPPORT YOU?"
is the best thing you can ask
when I hear these words
I'll answer and drop my mask

I can tell you I'm hurting
or I need some space
to simply back off
or to gladly embrace.

The Light Inside the Shadow

To You Who Has Never Known Depression, This Is My Gift (Silenus)

You say to me "why don't you just snap out of it?"
My initial reaction is, I'm used to hearing this shit.
But you showed concern, and a need to understand,
And that makes me want to stay my angry hand.

You told me that I always wallow, trapped in thought,
And I tell you that it's a trap in which I'm caught.
You suggest I should just get out and do some exercise,
I try to explain to you that my mind tells believable lies.

I tried to explain it to you, and my terminology was flawed,
I can see the iciness of your logic has not yet thawed.
So I plumb the depths of my experience, searching for common ground,
Reaching for a way to explain the rules by which I'm bound.

The only way I can think of to explain it is this,
And believe me, I am not taking the piss,
But there are chemicals flowing in our brains,
That steer our pleasures and direct our pains.

In part we are slaves to this ebb and flow,
And sometimes there's nowhere else to go,
No matter how much we wish it to be,
We cannot open the door with the key.

For six months I was a slave to my blanket and pillow,
And each moment trapped, I wanted to bellow,
I wanted to see it as simply as you,
And stop bubbling in this eternal stew.

But no matter how much I reached for a way out,
My mind was too clever, and continued this bout,
I wish I could tell you how difficult it's been,
But unless you've felt it, it's a sight unseen.

The word "depressed" is so often used,
I'm a little bit down, so this term I'll abuse,
But depression is so much more than just a slight hitch,
It's life hitting you full in the face, and life's a bitch.

We use that term "depression" in such an offhand way,
And it loses its power to explain its sway,
We aren't just making it up on the spot,
And can't just step away from the illness we've got.

So now I try to explain this great mess,
And I have no promises I'll succeed, I confess,
But nothing ventured, nothing gained,
And by the end, you may understand why I'm pained.

I know you understand physical ills and pains,
Like diabetes, MS, heart attacks and strains,
But you have to realise the same rules apply
To our brains and our thoughts, and they make us fry.

So now I try to explain it this way,
And believe me, I understand all that you say,
We should be able to just snap out of it and deal,
But it takes more than sane thought to make us heal.

All of the hopes and wishes in the world,
Can't begin to express how I want to be hurled
Out of the darkness and into the light,
But sometimes I have no energy to fight.

Most of the time, I function just fine,
But there's times when I'm lost and I cross the line,
It's not like I picked this future for me,
And it's not all that I hoped that I would be.

But here's the way that I try to impress
The way in which it's not just mild stress,
There's so much more to it than a bit of a down,
A mild heartache or the hint of a frown.

It sucks your life from out of your veins,
And I cannot begin to explain the pains,
For every moment is like your last,
And nothing exists, no future, no past.

You cannot see even a hint of light,
And believe me, this gives you an almighty fright,
And I hear you say, once again,
Get some exercise, and ease your pain.

The Light Inside the Shadow

I am trying so hard to bridge the gap,
And I don't want to place this pain in your lap,
But you have to see that we can't always understand,
That fate has dealt some of us a nasty hand.

Believe me, I have it within me to change,
But it's not always so simple or within my range,
I've tried just about everything under the sun,
And believe me I'm not doing this because it's fun.

It's taken me a long time to reach this point,
And I don't want to put your nose out of joint,
But f**k you if you judge me with a limited view,
Without first trying to understand what I've been through.

I want to hold up my hand just now,
And take a moment's pause to allow
You to take a while to think,
Because I've brought you to the brink.

I challenged you just now, and it wasn't just fun,
Because I need you to see the race that I've run,
Honestly, I'm smart, so surely you see,
If there was an easy way out, I'd have found it for me.

So now I come back to how to explain,
The pain that I suffer, how I feel my life drain,
It's not just a poetic device for effect,
This life can be truly and utterly fecked.

Well, now I'd like to set science's scene,
There's serotonin, melatonin and dopamine,
And lots of other brain chemicals,
That control our moods as basic animals.

Guess what? You can't always control your moods,
It's not like you've got a handle on your attitudes,
Depression is just like if someone "normal" is feeling low,
Except perhaps for the depths to which I go.

Just think for a minute how wonderfully it teased,
When in post-coital bliss you felt so pleased,
Well guess what, this is just you being a slave,
To the chemicals in your brain to which you cave.

The Light Inside

The same thing is true for me in my plight,
Struggling to see a moment of daylight,
Just as powerful chemicals are having their way,
And causing my basic emotions to sway.

So next time you think you understand this shit,
Take a look at the multitude of people who quit
This life, giving up the ultimate prize,
With no light of joy in their eyes.

It's not just having a bit of a rough day,
And it sure ain't saying it's tough but I'm okay,
The only difference between you and me,
Is the ups and downs go so much further, you see.

There's this wonderful thing called reality,
We filter it through our senses, what we hear and see,
But at the end of the day, it's just thoughts in our head,
And believe me, those thoughts can cause tears to be shed.

It would be so wonderful if we could just say stop,
And the streams of our thoughts would listen to this traffic cop,
But as much as we may want it to ease,
Sometimes our depression doesn't want to please.

Don't think for a minute I want this crap,
I've tried so much to give myself a slap,
But what is so damn easy for you,
Is sometimes something beyond what I can do.

So please take a minute to understand,
I've done my best through my times most bland,
I've hurt so much and not let it show,
But every now and then, I'm ready to blow.

But I've gotten to a point of wisdom, I think,
And this was learned at the edge, by the brink,
I've stopped seeing my down as my enemy,
And see it now as an essential part of me.

Depression is certainly not my enemy,
That's something that took me a long time to see,
In fact, it's a basic, fundamental part of me,
And I doubt, given the choice, I would want to be free.

The Light Inside the Shadow

It flows from the same source, so I see,
And gives me the great gift of creativity,
My hurt has made me feel so much more,
And it can lift me up or drag me to the floor.

But you have to understand a simple thing,
I don't always have the power to bring
Light to my life when all is dark,
And it's not because I want to be stark.

Sometimes my balance is just out of whack,
And your simple logic and solutions don't open a crack,
So just be patient, even though you may not understand,
I may be down, but I'd appreciate a hand.

Mental Illness: The Butterfly's Thoughts (TheBeautifulBlueButterfly)

We can see mental illness in so many ways.
It does not need to be too scary to talk about.
It does not need to be swept under the rug.
It is just like any other illness, disorder or disease.
It just happens to be that we cannot see it, but we feel it because it is there and it is real.

Sometimes we can control our emotions, sometimes we can tell ourselves to be strong and hang on there all by ourselves.
But other times we crash and burn and it is then that we need your help.

My ex boss thought I was making this up... Seriously mate, who wants to make that stuff up? If I could make this into fantasy instead of reality, I would. Oh how much easier it would be if this wasn't real, if this didn't exist. How much easier it would be if it was just some made up story that I'm not really a part of. How could you even think that I was using my illness as a crutch, as a scape goat?

Here's an idea...

Maybe if we get enough support around us, maybe we could all be great successes.
Maybe that boss could swallow his ignorance.
Maybe we could all raise a little awareness.

Maybe if we work ourselves out now, in the years to come we could be so much better. And if we're better, what we give to the world will be so much better quality.

So maybe we need to be selfish RIGHT NOW.
Get down and work ourselves out.
Go back to therapy and make myself "as better as I can be".
Do like the Ani DiFranco song and "Start on the inside and work your way out".

Author's Note: I have written/posted this piece to show my view of BiPolar and mental illness in general.

Stigma (creative)

Stigma for being different in a way is part of the "ingroup-outgroup" dynamic that you will find in all cultures, and is probably pre-human. It is an instinctual way of bolstering a group by excluding the other.

This is a good survival mechanism in a pre-industrial society, but very damaging in our complex culture as it is today. The only sane, constructive way to look at human differences and disabilities of any kind, including mental disorders, is this: "We are all from the Rift Valley in Africa." The ingroup is all of humanity.

People construct the outgroup by depersonalizing. We see Them as inferior, evil, less than ourselves.

A better attitude is that everyone has strengths and weaknesses. Also, strength can actually come from a perceived weakness. For example a perceived weakness of susceptibility to depression and bipolar disorder II has goaded me to develop empathy, compassion and the passion to fight injustice. These strengths give me immense satisfaction in helping to relieve suffering in others. If I didn't have this perceived weakness I wouldn't have the strength.

Some of the greatest artists and musicians of all time could well have been diagnosed as weak, schizophrenics, bipolar, or suffering from a personality disorder if they'd been in a different place and time. It was precisely their different ways of thinking and feeling that led to their greatness.

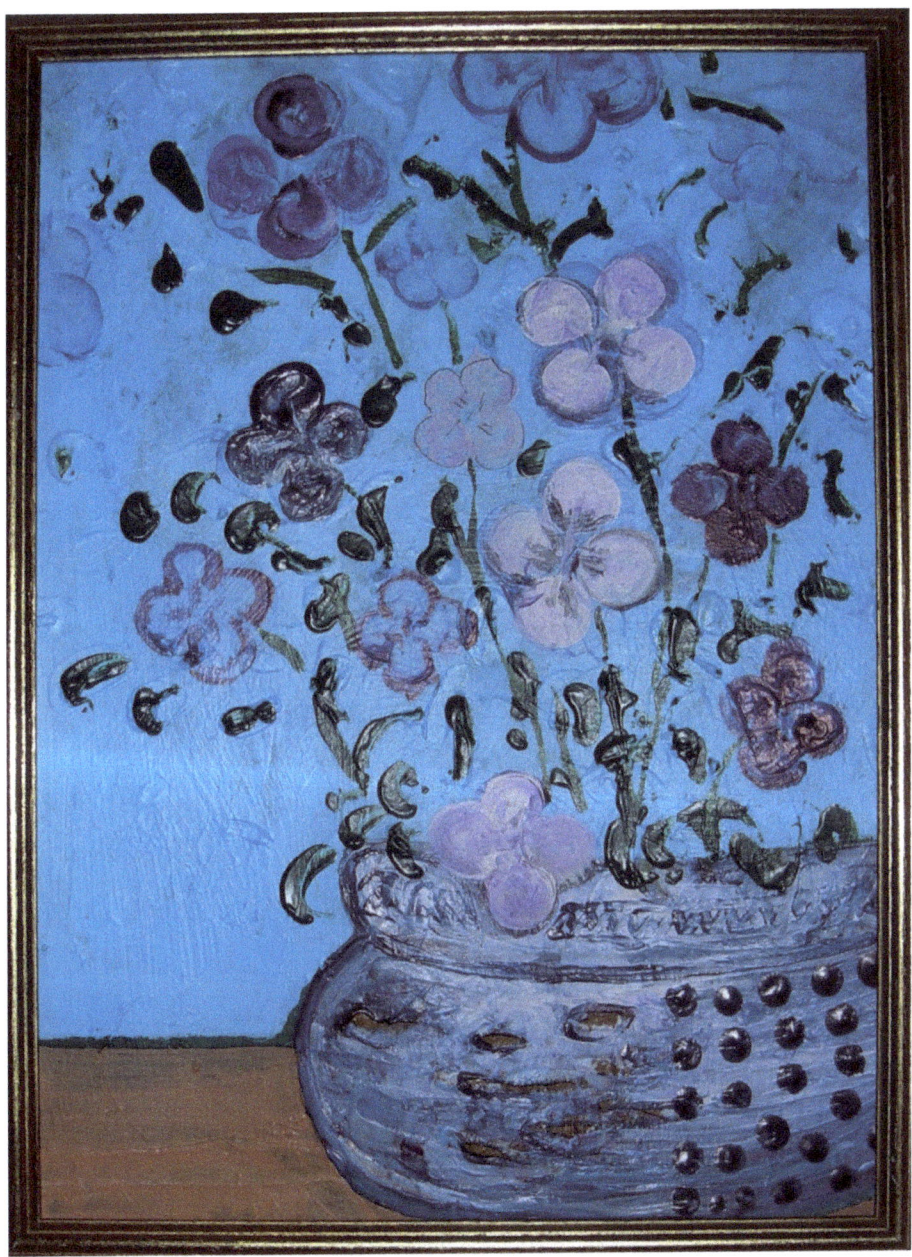

yesterday, today, tomorrow (creative)

'Yesterday, today and tomorrow' is the name of this particular plant which has flowers of three different colours: purple, blue and white. The Latin name of this plant is Brunfelsia Australis. It is also symbolic of the constant problem that people with mental disorders have, constantly thinking about the past the present and the future.

The Light Inside the Shadow

Eight Legs, Silk, Water and Light (Silenus)

I woke this morning, full of dread,
My inner demons, playing with my head,
They ripped at me, their talons cruel,
I considered hiding, a poor scared fool.

But something stopped me from playing dead,
And I rose from the comfort of my bed,
Dressed and ate my morning gruel,
Then entered my garden's morning cool.

I sat on a rock, waiting for who knows what,
Not really caring for life one jot,
And as I waited, lo and behold,
Something caught my eye, and it was gold.

The sun was shining, not yet hot,
I focused on this thing, within eyeshot,
I watched transfixed, this thing unfold,
This natural wonder, both subtle and bold.

The light was shining oh so bright,
And the angle there was just so right,
I caught my breath, and stared in wonder,
It stopped my world from tearing asunder.

A spider's web, so fragile and light,
Studiously built the previous night,
And here was I, in my morning blunder,
Trying to stop myself from going under.

The morning dew, wet and pendulous,
Hung from silky strands, fey and fabulous
The morning light, full of promise,
Caught my eye with visual bliss.

The spider caught me with its stimulus,
I stopped for a moment, feeling tremulous,
Nature, I realised, is oh so flawless,
And I gathered strength from seeming weakness.

Eight legs, silk, water and light,
Who'd have thought it would end my night?
Such simple parts that make a whole,
Warmth for my heart, salve for my soul.

A Poem (creative)

The pains and joy impart upon my world,
A dim glow soon contrasted by a turbulent blaze
gives me a chance to view the depths of men.
With uneventful simplicity
I breathe grandeur from the Earth
and I perceive above the norm.

Not unfair, this life,
if pain leads to the light.
For despite the dim
the wonder is there
to capture my curiosity
to inspire my soul.

Lost between fantasy and life
the wisdom is always there;
though twisted in misery and wonder
there is fire in my mind
not destructive but creative.

Colour my days, my months and my years
transparent and bright,
clear and vibrant.
The rainbow is always present
to warm, to inspire
the life lived on a razor's edge.

Coca Cola consciousness
lived in a Microsoft world
transformed by the Light
to reach the farthest heart.

Amongst the iPhone generation
I live my days in private
with uneventful simplicity.
I look at myself
the shadow of a man
who lives in a troubled world.

The Light Inside the Shadow

Reincarnated (GonePirate)

if reincarnation is the truth of it
I'll come back as a snake for the venom I spit
poison flooded out of my mouth like a river
a system for my toxins to deliver
but if it's true I'll just rot in hell
then that would really suit me well
I love to suffer for pain is home
and misery is all I've known
it's made me vicious vile as well
what of me, only time will tell
maybe I'll come back as a bird and fly
over your head into the sky
come back once to say goodbye
before I stay up so high
or more likely bound in a cage
filled with such a familiar rage
locked up imprisoned never to be free
another life that seems to suit me
maybe I'll come back as an ocean fish
this could be of what I wish

love the ocean love the sea
this seems to be the life for me
living in the water totally free
fills my fins with a sense of glee
then a shark comes along and gobbles me down
then my corpse will never be found
maybe I should be a shark turn the situation around
another life that makes me feel sound
killer of the sea a beast so deadly
another life that seems to please me
an animal bloodthirsty and hungry

but I know after this life there is nothing left
I died once when I ran out of breath
opened my eyes and I could see death
nothing to see but blackness
it's a sad truth that I have known
every living creature on this earth dies alone
and I don't say that in a morbid tone
I say that with a voice like stone
my life is mine for my own self
wouldn't put my pain on anyone else

full of life now that's real wealth
so here's to me and my good health
and may I live forever
I may not have it all together
but any storm I'll weather
giving up never

Jack was a homeless man (creative)

Jack was a homeless man
he lived in a wonderland
where love was all around him...

Jack was a story teller
a poet of the streets
where dreams kept him alive...

And he sang
songs of peace
and he played
a sad guitar
and he told me
he had a daughter
who he hadn't
seen for years

Jack was a friend of mine
I kept him company
through his hardest times...

Jack was an architect
who lost everything
when depression struck

And he told me
he had learned
through the suffering
he had grown
and he said
with a smile

Love is everything
love is all I need
love will stay with me
love will see me through

w.ingramcontent.com/pod-product-compliance
tning Source LLC
mbersburg PA
W041141170426
00CB00022B/2988